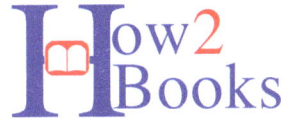

Giving you some ideas, do you want to know more?

Discover your Emotional Intelligence

Discover your Ikigai!

Getting to know your Biological, Physiological & Psychological SELF.

Relationships matter.

Relationships are important.

Building relationships.

Refresh your relationship.

Work through a damaged relationship.

Enrol in our course. Building life skills that will support you in your relationships.

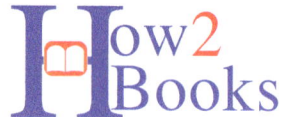

The book's main objective is to awaken the emotional intelligence and to give each reader, the quality of SELF and the value that should be placed on their individuality as a person and within their relationships.

Christine

Teacher of Psychology
Dip Ed, BA Ed, MACEA
CPD ACCREDITED

If you would like to study with us at Full Potential Education & Training and would like to undertake the Online Course, please contact:

>admin@fullpotentialtraining.com.au

This book brings to its readers the biological, physiological, and psychological approaches that connect to each person's emotional intelligence.

SEX SEXUALITY & RELATIONSHIPS

IT'S ALL ABOUT THE BIRDS AND THE BEES....!

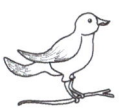 

This is not a medical resource book and should not be used as such. It is however a book for reference to each person's behaviour and their behaviour towards other people. The book gives an insight into how your human body, brain, hormones, and body chemistry work when you are in or about to go into a relationship.

If you have purchased this book without its cover, it may be stolen.

Neither the publisher nor the author is under any obligation to provide professional services in any way, legal, health or in any form which is related to this book, its contents or otherwise.

The laws and practices vary from country to country and state to state.

If legal or professional information is required, the purchaser or the reader should seek the information privately and best suited to their needs, and circumstances.

The author and publisher specifically disclaim any liability that may be incurred from the information within this book.

All rights reserved. No part of this book, including the interior design, images, cover design, diagrams, or any intellectual property (IP), icons, and photographs may be reproduced or transmitted in any form by any means (electronic, photocopying, recording, or otherwise) without the prior permission of the publisher. ©

Copyright© 2024 MSI Australia

All rights reserved.

ISBN:978-0-6459680-2-6

Published by How2Books
Under license from MSI Ltd, Australia
Company Registration No: 96963518255
NSW, Australia

See our website: www.how2books.com.au
Or contact by email: sales@how2books.com.au
Covers and Copyright owned by MSI, Australia

MSI acknowledges the author and images, text, and photographs used in this book.

(Re-edited copy, 2024)

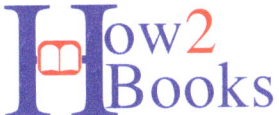

10% of the sale of each book helps to support Diabetes Type One and Cancer Research.

THE REASON WHY?

As the author of many books, over sixty have been written and published most with an emphasis on building life skills, health, and wellbeing. I too, until recently, have missed writing about our behaviour and our human sexuality!

Our human sexuality is as much a part of the topics listed above as any other human behaviour we care to speak about.

Having, in 2023, published four books for children and teens on puberty and a later book for parents on the process of hormone changes, as our children enter and go through puberty, all within the same year, it is only right to continue the conversation with this latest book on our human sexuality and the acts of love we have with our partners.

Let's get one thing right at the beginning, sexual activity is not bad or negative behaviour if the act is done with respect, care, and the love of another human being.

The act of sex should only be performed by two consenting adults and that is only when the act of intimate, and sexual touching should take place.

You will read the short story of a friend who, after her marriage broke down, had many one-night stands, and a one-night stand is no different to any other human act, it should be done with care, love and respect for the person or people involved.

Just recently, I did a little bit of editing for a friend who wants to write and is writing a book. I do not take on other people's writing, and I am not a ghostwriter, but I agreed to help as this person wanted desperately to start a novel. The novel has some sentences that lead to the sexual behaviour of a young couple, and as I read through the information, it seemed to me, that in that instance, the moments of intimacy were missing and even skirted around which made the wording written somewhat boring!

I started to add my own words, which to my surprise were different in connotation and meaning; I was truly getting into the way our human minds and bodies respond when we either fall in love or are attracted to different people as we go through life.

Our lives may have many different journeys, and when on those journeys, we meet different people, some we are attracted to and some not so! As I thought through the whole experience of writing for another person, and in the same week, going to the doctor about my health, during the appointment, the doctor and I spoke about relationships and how indeed, sex is good to have and good to enjoy, it is after all part of the glue that keeps relationships together and the community functioning.

And this is the reason why, and with the above thoughts and experiences, I now have written this book on sexual behaviour and the intimacy of relationships!

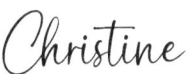

ONLINE, INDIVIDUAL COURSE

When a book is written, I always think, how would this book go in an online education package for my readers?

As a professional, accredited educator having graduated from the University of Canberra, Australia with a major in Psychology, Education is never far from my mind!

It is this insatiable drive that pushes me to give my readers the best information I can research and then form the hypothesis for writing a book.

We are all living in a world of uncertainty and the more life skills we each independently learn and develop, the safer, we not only keep ourselves but also our loved ones, family, friends, and communities.

Well-informed information helps in the structure of relationships, the security of SELF, and the cohesion of communities. This is why when we each use the tools that individual emotional intelligence offers, we grow, extend our learning capacity, and flourish in all that we do and can accomplish.

To support you in a deeper understanding of how your mind and body work; you will need to understand how your Biology, Physiology, and Psychology work within your relationships.

The 8 Module online, individual course is now ready and available and, once bought, can be downloaded to your computer.

CHAPTERS	PAGE
CHAPTER ONE What is sex?	2
CHAPTER TWO What is sexuality?	20
CHAPTER THREE What does sexuality include?	34
CHAPTER FOUR Fascination hormones...!	64
CHAPTER FIVE Let's talk about sex hormones!	89
CHAPTER SIX Understanding sex: the male and female body	105
CHAPTER SEVEN Relationships	137
CHAPTER EIGHT The Ikigai in Each of Us...	169
OTHER BOOKS WRITTEN By Christine Thompson-Wells	175

WHAT IS SEX?

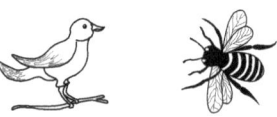

A PERSONAL NOTE

This book is meant to open the conversation!

Many people may feel uncomfortable when speaking about sex, sexuality, and relationships. However, these subjects play a critical role in your life.

Communities across the world, through either cultural, psychological, religious, and or philosophical, may consider the topics to be taboo, and yet, speaking about the above subjects will improve people's lives, add great value to individual well-being and health, and limit areas of crime that grow through this lack of knowledge.

CHAPTER ONE
What is sex?

When two or more people have natural intimacy, which is a means of physical and emotional pleasure, contributing to human bonding and/or reproduction.

Sexual intercourse between a male and female (binary relationship[1]) is a human activity involving the thrusting of the male penis inside the female vagina; it is a natural human behaviour for human beings to have sex, and indeed nearly all living organisms...!

Or when physical pleasure and enjoyment, and is, in equal participation. As with all information that contains taboo words or suggestions, the earlier in the conversation those words or suggestions are mentioned, the easier the flow of conversation becomes in the future!

---

[1] PLEASE NOTE: Not all people identify as binary in the traditional sense of male and female. There are many different relationships that exist beyond binary.

How To Create a Sexual and Loving Relationship

Now we have those two first paragraphs out of the way, let's get on with the rest of the book...!

Without sex, and or mating happening on the planet, all living creatures, great and small, would have become extinct millions of years ago or they and us would never have materialised anyway...!

According to the researcher, Joann Rodgers, Director of Media at Johns Hopkins Medical Institute has said about human sexual activity, *"People and indeed all animals are hard-wired and will continue to do so,"* Rodgers said in a recent interview. *"I imagine that this evidence shows that people at least like sex and even if they don't, they engage in it as a biological imperative. "*

Further research through the Dark Ages reveals, *"The low priority attached to sexual pleasure by people who lived in distant times is inexplicable unless one considers the hindrances that existed in those days,"* Shorter, a researcher, writes and identifies, "*...especially to the 1,000 years of misery and disease—often accompanied* *by some very un-sexy smells and itching—that led up to the Industrial Revolution. After the mid-nineteenth century, these hindrances start to be removed, and the great surge towards pleasure begins.* "

In this book, we are talking about our human natural behaviour, not the behaviour of any other organism. Sex is an extremely wide subject and involves many cultures, religions, faiths, historical facts and of course, human behaviour. Having sex falls into the category of psychology and is within those activities, each being a fundamental part of that subject.

In biological terms, we humans sit within the term of placental mammals. The placenta forms in the early embryonic stage of the development of the foetus. This placenta is rich in nutrition which helps to ensure the best possible outcome for the child once it is born.

Now that we know the above, we are ready to speak about the sexually performing adult.

HISTORICAL FACTS

GERMANY

In 2008, a phallic representation of a penis was found at Hohle Fels, Germany, and dates back twenty-eight thousand years. It is thought to be the oldest representation of a phallus to date. Like so many phalli it may represent, not sex as we know it in our modern day, but as a monument to fertilisation of the soil for good harvest or as a symbol of future life! Of course, we will never understand the true meaning of this phallus, but it gives us a general idea of how people were thinking so many years ago...!

ANCIENT ISRAEL

Neolithic images of female genitalia, between seven to nine thousand years old, have been found in Southern Israel. The stones clearly show the opening of the female vaginal area. They may be symbolic and have ritualistic meanings encouraging good harvests.

EGYPT

Sexual representation was an important part of Egyptian society. The phallus played a role in the cult of Osiris in ancient Egypt. When Osiris was murdered, his body was cut into many parts, his wife retrieved the parts, but the penis was missing. She had a wooden, erect penis, (phallus), made and secured it to the found body parts. Osiris was believed to be the god of fertility.

ANCIENT GREECE AND ROME

Moving on, having said the above, ancient Rome had a different slant on sex which has been revealed in the digs of, and around Pompeii, and Herculaneum, both covered by ash and pumas during the eruption of Mount Vesuvius in 79AD. The ash and pumas have indeed preserved many buildings, frescoes, artifacts, and household items decorated with sexual themes. Such findings show the natural relationship the residents may have had with the natural functioning of the human bodies of both males and females!

Another Roman significance to the phallus was the winged phallus which denoted the magical or mystical deities that had significance for the people of the time.

Romans, and Greeks, decorated houses, public baths, and public places with impressions of penises. Other significant actions relate to the value of the human genitals, for example, while swearing an oath, Hebrews, Romans, Egyptians, and Semitic Arabs had a custom of holding their crotch!

Eroticism may have come into the thinking of the artists of the time as they developed many forms of art. Eroticism may have been part of everyday thinking and behaviour, and culturally based on the value and belief systems of the residents of Pompeii and Herculaneum where the sculpture of the god Pan performing sex with a goat was discovered. Of course, today, we frown on and try not to think about such human activities!

Other artifacts have been discovered during the digs which suggest the erect penis found on a clay tablet may have been to encourage good harvest or rainfall for the region.

ROME AND GREECE – FEMALE FORM

Also seen on a circular plaque from the ancient Roman and Greek eras shows three female volvas and a winged phallus. This may be a ritualistic symbol or some type of sign suggesting sexual pleasure and intimacy!

ANCIENT INDIA

The god Shiva is one of the widely worshipped male deities of India. The lingam (which is the representation of a male erect penis), dates to prehistoric times. Lingams are found in many ancient temples and displayed in museums. The essence of the teaching of Hinduism is that of respect for life, all living things, and the earth on which we all live.

Historical fact shines a light on the thoughts of the writers of the Kamasutra, an ancient Sanskrit text of India. The text, possibly first written around four hundred BCE, outlines sexual movements which allow for sexual achievement, eroticism, and personal fulfilment.

The philosophy describes the love of life and the appreciation of love and passion. The script signifies the Principles of Love and speaks of the movements that allow for sexual satisfaction, and personal pleasure, combined with body contentment. Above all else, it is the respect for the human body, mind, and soul of the relationship of the people within the lovemaking of the moment, and the reverence of the time spent.

INTERPRETATION OF THE FOUR MAIN GOALS OF THE KAMASUTRA

DHARMA relates to good behaviour, moral rights, and the management of social order.

ARTHA relates to the 'means of life,' which incorporates wealth, career, financial security, and prosperity.

KAMA relates to passion, emotions, the pleasure of the senses, enjoyment and satisfaction of life, love, sexual activities, moral responsibility, spiritual liberation and more.

MOKSHA relates to liberation or the release from the cycle of death and rebirth, self-knowledge, self-realisation, and freedom.

(If this philosophy interests you, please research more.)

INDONESIA

Many cultures adopt different customs. Accordingly, Prince Puger achieved kingly and higher powers when swallowing semen from the phallus of an already dead sultan.

BHUTAN

The phallus is often seen in paintings, carved in wood and the end tied with a white ribbon. These are secured to the doorways of houses to ward off evil spirits.

ANCIENT SCANDINAVIA

This is the land of my ancestors, and the phallus is too, part of traditional beliefs. The Nordic god Freyr represented a phallic deity of male fertility and love.

SWEDEN

The Cobbler, a Bronze Age, (1700-500BCE), is one of several rock carvings found in the Lysekil Municipality. The Cobbler shows an extended penis which may relate to the Weather god, a predecessor of Thor. The Cobbler has both arms and hands raised with the hammer appearing close to his reach!

IRAN

In Khaled Nabi cemetery, Iran, the dead are remembered by the representation of phallic tombstones which may give the suggestions of pre-Islamic fertility cults.

JAPAN

During a warring uprising of 1467-1603, the ruler Yoshitaka, was forced to commit ritual suicide. The son of the ruler, once found, was murdered and his penis was cut into small pieces. Out of respect for the boy, the villagers built a monument which is surrounded by numerous large phalluses. Today, it is a tourist destination where people can rub a phallus, pray, and ask for success in fertility, love, vitality, and marriage.

BALKANS

Around the year, 3,000BCE, Kukeri existed; the Kukeri were described as a divinity. Now, and as part of the Balkan tradition, the Kukeri have become a part of Balkan annual culture. During the festival, the Kukeri are seen dressed in a goat or sheep pelt, wearing a horned mask, and girded with a large wooden phallus. The annual festival identifies the toiling in the fields, the fertilisation of women partners and the trauma and pain of childbirth.

SWITZERLAND

The Swiss bear on the Swiss coat of arms is seen carrying a log; according to tradition, the log was once a phallus. Originally, the log was painted bright red and represented penises. The red, erect painted penis is still seen on the bear, as he walks, but is minus the testicles!

THE AMERICAS

The Mayan culture represented the male penis in both stone wall carvings and in many sculptures of phalli. In pre-Columbian America, the Mayans identified the Tonsured Maize god which also represents fertility.

ENGLAND

England is not renowned for its phallus in stone carvings or decorative wall embellishments of phallus, but King Henry VIII is known for wearing exaggerated codpieces when posing for painting or when he was in his grand attire. So, what is a codpiece? A codpiece is a triangular piece of fabric that was used to cover a man's fly in the fifteenth and sixteenth centuries. In many of Henry VIII portraits, the King stands proud emphasizing the large codpiece which was meant to identify his strength in producing male heirs, protection of the country and other male or ruler attributes. The codpiece is further exaggerated when seen in the King's armour, displayed as a bulbous codpiece way beyond the natural size of what was needed….!

How To Create a Sexual and Loving Relationship

CHRISTIANITY

Humans, when in happy and loving relationships, from the beginning of time, through the last three hundred thousand years, have liked to enjoy sex. It is a natural need of the biological body to feel someone else or to feel and be touched by another person.

When Christianity, and indeed, other religious philosophies, entered people's lives, much of the natural touching may have been removed from and within relationships! Yes, there have always been pockets in society that resist and do not follow strict religious boundaries, but for many people caught up in different religious doctrines, the freedom of the spirit and movement were restricted, and the tightness of the teachings may have contributed to great stress and strain within people's lives.

Respect is fundamental to all relationships, but for good health and well-being, humans need to be able to freely live and enjoy each moment as it happens.

VICTORIAN ERA

'With the rapid advancement of industrialisation, there appeared to be a decrease in morality and personal values...!' Well, that was the idea of the ruling class of the Victorian era in the United Kingdom and other Western-thinking countries! In just one instance, it was considered scandalous for a woman to show any part of her skin, all body parts had to be covered, apart from her face...! If a woman showed her ankle, it was considered, she had little virtue and was possibly tantamount to a hussy!

With such strict clothing codes, codes of conduct and other restrictive codes which led to strict attitudes, it placed intolerable restrictions on people's lives. Such attitudes and codes restricted freedom of expression, thus, creating a culture of conformity! Conformity stifles creative invention, imagination, self-expression, and uniqueness!

Within many of the attitudes, still in some individual thoughts and ideas that people have in the twenty-first century; assumptions of other people are often made. Many assumptions have residue conditioning of the Victorian era! Often, assumptions are outdated and do not have substance, but the judgement of another person is made, and the sentence is passed. Such pre-conditioning of attitudes from the Victorian era often happens in families, communities and indeed in countries around the world!

So, sex is about people coming together to enjoy the natural flow of their bodies in movement, feelings, passion, and love. Sex is a natural function of the human body which adds wellness, good mental health, and the passion to live each day to its full potential.

Sex is about giving to another the enjoyment of the body, the satisfaction that what is happening between the people taking part is of good meaning and intention. Sex is not just for one participating partner but for both. Good sex takes time, love, and an intimate understanding of each other's needs.

Not all sex meets the full orgasmic state because people are sensitive to their feelings, the worries of the day, and other life considerations. Keeping this in mind, the act of sex needs to be done with care, love, sensitivity, and thought.

YOUR THOUGHTS

How To Create a Sexual and Loving Relationship

WHAT IS SEXUALITY?

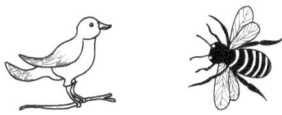

CHAPTER TWO
What is sexuality?

When we identify with the way we think and the types of partners we want in our lives, we are working with our sexuality. It may take many years for some people to find the partner that is right for them!

Each person's sexuality is important and needs to be respected. Being young and living in a world of ever more changing attitudes can become difficult for many young people as they go through the passages of life from the child to teen and then into adulthood. Each one of these passages is a rite of passage and should be understood. Each baby born will go through the rites of passage that allow them to become adults.

Not all rites of passage are easy and some, because of heritage, different living environments, misunderstood role models, and other complications a young person experiences, can lead to difficulties in understanding their own and private sexuality. Once a person has come to grips, that there are many different people in the world, and each person contributes their uniqueness to the community in which they live, life can become all-embracing and full of purpose.

Understanding sexuality is diverse because of the many types of sexuality each person has either adopted or their sexuality is part of their personality. Each person may think, 'This is my sexuality...' but over time, sexuality may change, and that same person may feel different about their sexuality as time passes and in the years that follow.

Coming to terms with your sexuality can be a positive, liberating, and a time of mentally growing and maturing into the person, you are meant to be. Whilst, you are changing with every new experience, with each experience, the personal growth undertaken can add to the rich fabric of life.

Creating and wanting positive outcomes in relationships is the mutual respect for a person or for the group you are choosing to belong to. Respect in all relationships cannot be underrated but must be a priority of every new relationship. If respect does not exist, (regardless of the emotions felt), the relationship will be fraught with danger, heartbreak, and despair.

There are no right or wrong ways about your sexuality, your sexuality is the way you are. Sadly, while many people are on their journey of discovery, if not familiar with real-life experiences, some people will take advantage of a person, (regardless of age), while that person is seeking to discover their sexuality, this is partly the reason for this book!

No person should be left in the wilderness because they are on a journey to find out their sexuality.

Young people are not unique in the search for identifying their sexuality, it may be a mother of a child or many children; it may be the man or woman that has been faithful and loyal in their marriage; it may be the man or woman who has not found true happiness or love in any of their previous relationships!

The doorway to open such a conversation can be vast, but it is a journey of discovery and if done honestly with care and love, many people can benefit from finding out about their sexuality.

Sexuality is not necessarily about who you have sex with, how often sex is performed, and other areas that are confused with the word sexuality. Your sexuality is about your sexual feelings, how attracted you are to other people, what you find interesting in people, and your behaviours toward different people! Sexuality is about how you feel emotionally and how you physically feel when you see other people. You may see a person, and have an instant attraction to that person, this is your sexuality coming into focus.

Whilst you may be attracted to another person, that person may not be attracted to you; this is all part of the sexuality that goes on in everyday life with millions of people worldwide.

It is the weaving of emotions that we experience different reactions to different people and situations that proves to be the learning that most people, who wish to grow, go through.

Many people in relationships, (married or otherwise), want to get to know different people outside of their established relationship! Whilst, this may be accepted by one partner, it may be rejected by another!

If a person is on a quest to identify, and this quest may come later in life, their unique sexuality, can lead to turmoil and confusion if not managed sensitively! In an established relationship, if the change is not managed with love and care, the change can be hurtful to the established partner or other people within the family or group involved.

Let's remember, this is your life, and you are on a mission to find out, 'who you are…!' There are ways of managing these situations, but it is important, that those people who are close to you, have feelings and the best way forward, is to sit and talk with those people you care about.

You are a person; you may be drawn to the opposite or same sex; each person relates to people differently. If the person you are drawn to, feels like the way you feel, and not all new relationships turn out to be sexual, but they may have a sexual overtone of care and love for another person, and this may be the groundwork for a deep and lasting friendship.

There are many forms of love, and each person has their guidelines, values, and rules. Each person you love will also have their guidelines for the way they want to spend time in a relationship. This is all part of sexuality and the way you love and care for your relationships.

How To Create a Sexual and Loving Relationship

Even the most committed and deep relationships do change over time. Values change, what was once a priority at the start of the relationship, may now be taking second or third place, this is all part of each person's individual growth and within all growth, there are renewal processes that can change the dynamics of the strongest relationships.

WHAT DOES SEXUALITY INCLUDE?

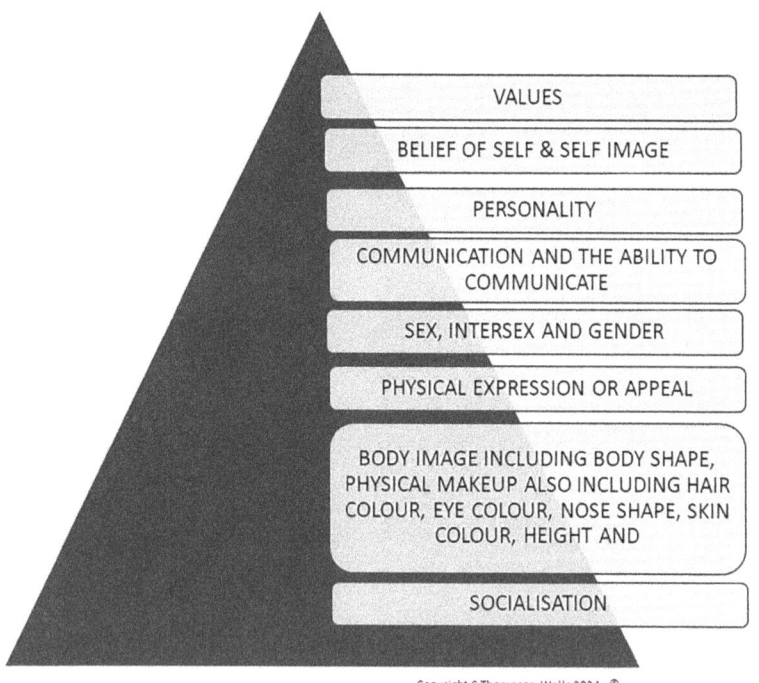

Copyright C Thompson-Wells 2024 ©

It is the combination of the opposite Personality Pyramid and many other features that are inherent within your makeup that create sexual attraction to other people, and to mention here, we may not be aware that we have these assets until one day, another person tells us 'Just how attractive we are…!' to them!

To many of us, this may come as a shock and a surprise, so don't ever underrate yourself…!

Now, let's take each of your assets one at a time!
✓ Talent

....

✓ Ability

....

✓ Skill/s

....

✓ Qualification/s

....

✓ Blessings

....

✓ Resources

....

✓ Experiences and more.

....

....

....

....

As you go through the chapters, you may want to record your thoughts to list aspects and assets of your personality in the boxes on the next page. Throughout your mind-work and note-taking, you may find that opinions, choices, and desires change. You may also find that your once firmly set ideas are starting to move and modify and your viewpoint is, indeed, different from previously!

Remembering here, that your ASSETS include your:
✓ The Biological
✓ The Physiological and
✓ The Psychological within SELF.

You are SELF. In adult sexual relationships, we are in control of SELF. We do not own or control other people. For a relationship to grow and advance, there needs to be balance and respect.

RELATIONSHIP DYNAMICS INCLUDE:
RESPECT
Within this seven-letter word, it has the following understanding built into it:

- ✓ Kindness
- ✓ Communication
- ✓ Unselfish love
- ✓ Compromise and fun or laughter.

Other considerations will include:

- ✓ Sensitivity for other people, their belongings, rights, and wishes.
- ✓ Care and regard include the valuing of another person or people within the group and or family and treating all with kindness.
- ✓ Understanding and impact, recognizing that all actions, including words spoken, have outcomes.

Understanding also relates to the dynamics of treating other people with empathy, which without, can and may cause distress or harm to another person.

- ✓ Avoiding harm and hurt is within the dynamic of RESPECT.
- ✓ Feeling safe and not in 'harm's way' allows for honesty and truthfulness within the relationship.
- ✓ Being patient while listening to another person's point of view is within RESPECT.
- ✓ RESPECT also implies, that dominance has no place within the relationship.
- ✓ Allowing each person to experience their own space when needed.

The understanding of RESPECT is a learned value and comes within the well-being of the relationship.

How To Create a Sexual and Loving Relationship

KEEPING YOU ON TARGET

As you start to look from the 'INSIDE OUT,' write down in the boxes below the assets you have. To give you an example, an asset is the value you cherish.

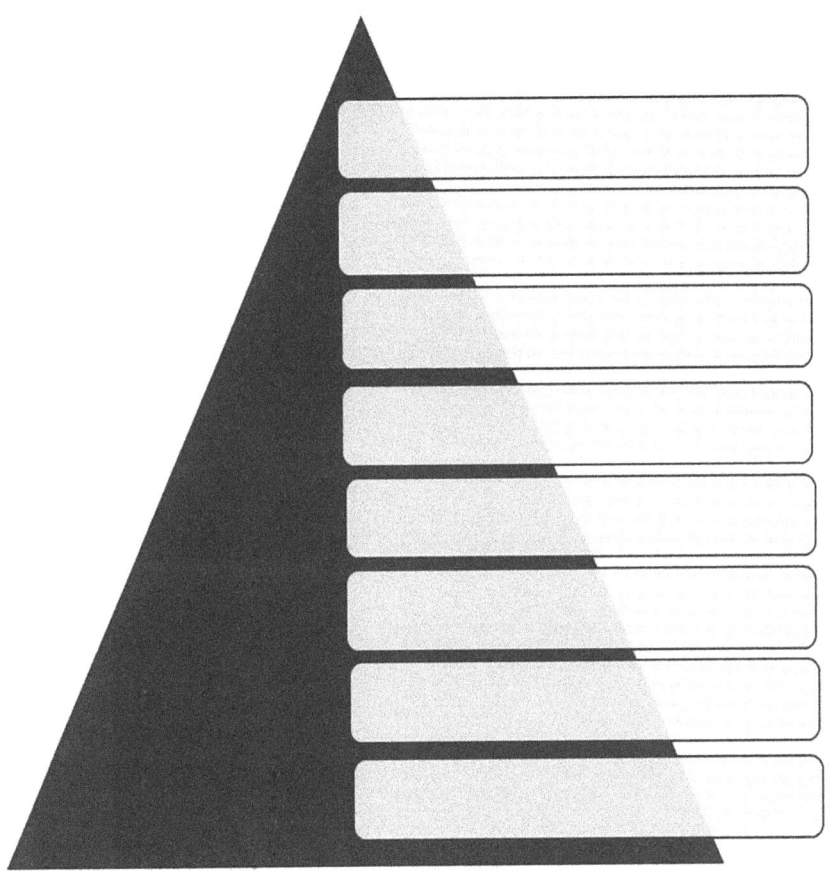

YOUR THOUGHTS

How To Create a Sexual and Loving Relationship

WHAT DOES SEXUALITY INCLUDE?

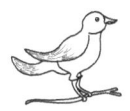 

CHAPTER THREE
What does sexuality include?

By taking one asset at a time, you can slowly work from the 'INSIDE OUT' which will help you to access further hidden assets; you are now on a journey of personal discovery.

VALUES

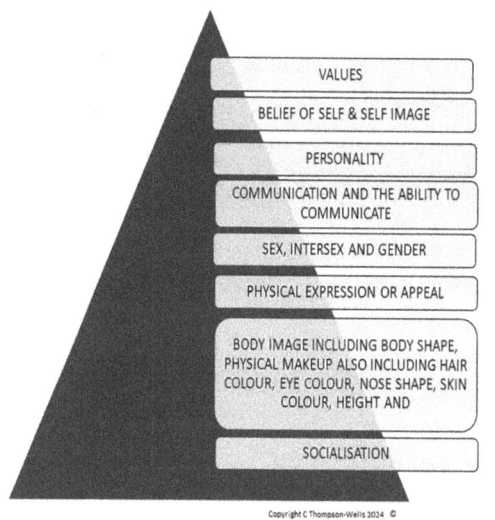

Each person has their value system and what is of value to one person, may not be of value to another!

Your values form part of your assets.

In every relationship, it is wise to take your time and not assume another person's values. Each value a person has is deeply rooted and may be inherent within their traits and personality.

(In the last chapter, I mentioned the word assumptions and the Victorian era, and now, I will expand on that word! Assumptions: other people's assumptions have got many innocent people into trouble; in times as recently as the sixteenth century, an assumption of another person had the victim burnt at the stake!)

Having said the above, we cannot assume anything about another person unless we take the time out to listen and get to know another person and understand their values!

With the past firmly in the past, we are fortunate, in many situations, to be born in the twentieth and twenty-first centuries where many different relationships form part of the community. Many people want to live differently, rather than in the conventional marriage, as in a man and woman, (heterosexual or binary[2]) relationship! Other people who don't want the conventional relationship, but may wish to live with their

---

[2] In social, cultural, and beliefs, binary is accepted as there are only two categories within human sexuality: male and female. In other words, a person is either masculine or feminine!

chosen partner, can, in many instances, freely live their lives as they wish! There are many exchanged and respected values that help to create many successful relationships.

To note here, if a person enters a relationship to change another person, they in many instances, may be wanting to interfere and want to change the values of that person! This type of intention is dishonest, and painful and can lead to long-term problems in the mental health of another person; this should not be the intention within any relationship!

WORKING WITH THE PERSONALITY PYRAMID AND YOUR VALUES
BELIEF IN SELF & SELF IMAGE
As we go through life there are rites of passage, each rite is a time that raises your awareness of the magnificence of your ability to achieve or aim for higher life goals.

Many rites of passage are linked to religious ceremonies as in the Jewish religion of circumcision of the male penis where the foreskin is removed from the outside of the penis; the ceremony, if a child is delivered naturally, and the child is well, takes place on the eighth day after birth!

The ceremony of marriage is a rite of passage, big 'O' birthdays are a rite of passage as in turning fifty or in other birthdays, as in turning eighteen, and twenty-one! The final 'rite of passage' according to the anthropologist, Elisabeth Kubler-Ross, is the rite of passage of dying!

Rites of passage, self-belief, and self-image are related to each other. Many rites of passage are linked to traditions and may be inherited and connected to your ancestry and your philosophy of life.

Many rites of passage are also linked to the goals you achieve. Regardless of how lofty many goals are, most are obtainable through work, dedication, and the desire to win that goal…!

When you write down a goal, you are indeed writing down a mental contract and mental contracts are extremely powerful tools when you want to reach goals or achieve milestones in your life. Two milestones that come instantly to mind are completing a university degree or building a home.

With accomplishing both above achievements there must be belief in yourself to complete all tasks that lead to the successful completion of the result.

Other goals may be to go into business for yourself or to learn a new skill, all can be done with the right mindset and the determination to win your goal.

Self-image is equally important. When facing and looking at self-image, you need to have respect firmly within your vision. Self-image drives many industries which include fashion, the fitness industry, and others, but if we go deeper than that, positive self-image is about self-respect and when you respect something, you treat it with reverence and admiration. Maintaining a positive self-image is important in maintaining your relationships.

With a positive self-image and when you were born, you came into the world as a new little person, you had all the DNA that would allow you to transition into a whole grown-up human being. It is the journey from birth to now, that forms the world views you have.

However, we need to pause at this point because there are often misunderstood ideas about new babies that come into the world!

Yes, because the child is new, and when looking into the eyes of a newborn, what is missing is the understanding, that this child has come into being, and the image we see has come down from generation to generation and each part of the child is an ancient part given to that child through the connection of two people having sex, making love or through other means such as in vitro fertilization (IVF).

The child may have the eyes of a distant, past grandparent, DNA parts of the heart, or intestines of another ancestor, so you should not assume that the child is completely new, it is a combination of ancient people that is brought together in one miracle at conception and this child was you.

So, keeping this complicated story in mind, you are the outcome that deserves a great deal of respect, from within your own, but ancient brain, and the knowledge that you are you.

With this knowledge you can tap into many talents and build skills from that talent, these skills are life skills and are meant to keep you safe, they are not only meant to keep you safe, but are meant to allow you to develop a particular specialist flair, capacity, or genius for building a secure base from which you can live your life.

You may find you are attracted to law, the arts, fashion, design, and finance or have a creative force where you can think 'outside the box,' and see there is a need in the community and fill that 'need' with a solution.

I have a friend who designed tactiles for use at curbs on the pavements, on railway stations, and stairs in public places; they are bright colours, yellow, blue, red, and so on. These tactiles are designed to keep people safe and to stop them from walking onto the road at the traffic lights; stop people from getting too close to the edge of the platform at railway stations; they are designed to stop accidents, while people do their jobs and live their daily lives. This is an example of a good and creative talent and thinking 'outside the box!' This talent may have its roots in past ancestry, but now in the twenty-first century has been put to good use.

The fact that somebody takes on the challenge to 'think outside the box...,' an onlooking person may find sexually attractive, another person may find this type of aspiration utterly frustrating...!

As you start to look at yourself from the 'INSIDE OUT' and not the outside in, you will start to see a new vision of yourself, and this new part is part of your sexuality that makes you a unique and different person from all the other people you may know!

PERSONALITY

We can each modify our personality. Like so many areas of your life, you can choose to work with a negative or positive personality. If you choose to be miserable, then that is the world you will live in – a miserable world of existence!

However, if you choose to have a positive personality, you can make even the toughest situations work for you.

To give you some idea, I once had a business, a flower shop, and a floristry school. I had trained as a florist in London in the sixties, it took five years to complete my training, it was tough, they were long days and all for thirty shillings a week! I was fifteen when I started this training. How I envied my friends who were working in warm offices and being paid five pounds a week and so many times, I just wanted to walk away from the 'so-called training' but something inside of me kept pushing me forward. It most definitely wasn't the sore fingers, the small wage but something so much deeper...!

Eventually, I had finished my training, and I was being paid eleven pounds a week, so much more money than any of my friends. In the end, I could run and manage a business, make wedding bouquets, and floral designs, manage staff, and teach the subject of commercial floristry. That skill has been a great benefit to my life, and it was the thought, 'Why do people buy flowers?' that sent me on to university, and still today, I have many questions that I'm still searching for answers about...! It was a tough five-year training, but through the experiences, I have built life skills and a means to self-sustainability.

It is managing the tough times in life that allow you to keep going and reach the goals you have set for yourself.

So, what is human personality? Human personality includes feelings, thoughts, and patterns of thoughts, behaviours, and outcomes. Outcomes are the results of different behaviours you have used or in different words said! It is sometimes easy to say something, and regret having said it! Often, in the heat of a discussion or argument, hurtful words are said, or hateful actions are taken. In many instances, it is at the end of a relationship that this negative and sometimes destructive side of your or our personality shows itself!

In most instances, if you cast your thoughts back to the beginning of the relationship, not a hurtful word was spoken, or a destructive action taken! It is the erosion of respect for another person that can bring to the surface retaliation for hurts received during a relationship! It is managing the hurts and experiences of the past relationship that prepares you for the next relationship.

When I've been in a long-term relationship and that relationship ends, I know from experience now, that it takes me from three to seven years to restore my emotions and to feel the readiness of a new relationship! Not everybody has this same experience, but I like to know that I am ready to restart my life with another person!

Your personality has many intricate parts and possibly too many to discuss in this book. Your personality, though in minor modification through life experiences, is possibly a constant and does not change a great deal as you journey through life!

Each person's personality is part of the integration of their psychological makeup, which would include, heritage, memories of visions of role models during childhood, culture, religious or faith backgrounds, and life experiences.

The physiology of a person also has a bearing on how a person's personality develops. When a person is given a challenge at birth as in being born with a disability, many young people take on the challenge to aspire and be the best they can be and to achieve their goals. We only need to look at young athletes who have challenges set before them to see the aspiration they bring into their lives in gaining entrance to the Olympics and other great feats they accomplish.

Taking on the challenge and achieving your goals allows you to feel accomplished and to be an independent thinker and action-taker.

From my own experiences, if I had listened to many people, including many family members, I would have stopped researching, writing books, and developing my publishing business. When you, or we, hear a negative comment that hurts your or our heart, and with me, it makes the challenge of accomplishment to reach my goals even stronger!

If people find what you are doing uncomfortable to recognize and accept, please remember, this is their uncomfortableness and not yours...!

Your determination may also contribute to your sex appeal, and your strength of character...

COMMUNICATION AND THE POWER TO COMMUNICATE
Communication is an ancient action that has been used throughout the evolution of, not only the human species but all animals, indeed, with all organisms who have a life and a commitment to meet their destiny! Someone or two-cell organisms may only exist to reproduce, but even in such a primitive one or two-cell state, each communicates to the other that there is mating to do! Communication between cells is called intercellular signalling and communication within a single cell is called intracellular signalling.

So, forms of different communication have been around ever since the single cell developed!

You may think, what has the above got to do with sexual relationships? It is the hidden or not verbally or physically transmitted communication from one person to another, possibly not initially recognised, that may initiate the start of a relationship...!

Developing communication skills takes time and persistence. Human communication is so much more complicated than in a one or two-cell organism, and this is why, the art of effective communication is important in all relationships, including intimate relationships with our partners! In some instances, your relationship with another person may be short, it may be one night, but during that interaction within that relationship, all passed and received communication needs to be understood!

It is often the unseen communication, the visual, non-spoken incoming information, the information, 'you cannot put your finger on...,' that gives you the knowledge that it is the start or end of a relationship!

Using the information that is medically defined:
SEX, INTERSEX, GENDER
Sex, intersex, and gender are topical issues in this current time. After writing the children and young adult

books on puberty, it is only natural to carry on the conversation.

SEX refers to the differences between males and females. Having previously mentioned, a male baby comes into being at about the eighth week after conception. It is the development of the XY chromosome that makes the difference in the sex of a male. Females are females from conception. Females have the XX chromosome.

Because of imaging and advanced technology, the sex of a child can be identified in the early stages of the pregnancy. The normal word 'sex' relates to what sex the child is, male or female!

Each person typically has their sex assigned at birth, this relates to their physiology including their genitalia, chromosomes[3], and hormone composition. Identification of the sex of a child at birth is known as 'natal sex.'

---

[3] Each cell is a molecule which contains a nucleus. The nucleus encloses a threadlike structure called a chromosome that contains DNA.

A female develops within the female womb because, within the formation of chemistry carried by the mother, there is the XX chromosome. While the XX chromosome is active, contained within the chemistry is the activation of hormones which include estrogen, progesterone, and some levels of testosterone. Females, like males, also have different levels, sometimes lower levels, of testosterone.

As said, the male baby carries the chromosomes XY and this makes the differences between the male and female binary. The male hormone testosterone is activated at about eight weeks which helps to trigger the development of the male penis and testicles.

The human baby comes into existence through the act of impregnation and the chemical makeup of human adults!

INTERSEX
When a baby is born, there may be a natural variation within the formation of their genitals. In some instances,

a baby may be born with sex organs that fall outside the male or female classifications as acknowledged in the binary description! An intersex baby may be born with both testicular and ovarian tissues or formations.

Being intersex is a naturally occurring variation of the chemistry taking place in the cell development of the child. The child can be biologically healthy but will have a different chromosome formation than the binary child born.

If the body of the baby is healthy and functioning properly, the choice of change is personal as the baby grows, develops, and goes into adulthood.

GENDER

There are many ways people may choose to define their gender, each is personal, and is part of the value system built into each person's personality.

Gender is an internal sense and awareness of self and how you, as an individual, want the world to see and acknowledge you; it is somewhat different from the term 'sexuality'.

Gender is how a person identifies, it is not necessarily made up within the binary views and exclusively the male or female outlook...!

A person who identifies themself as having a gender difference or spectrum is identifying themselves from an individual viewpoint or spectrum. Spectrums do vary and may include, transgender, nonbinary, intersex, gender neutral, genderfluid, and genderqueer among other identities.

When a person chooses to defend their gender, they do so through thoughts and making independent choices of how they want to be viewed or perceived in society. These choices meet the psychological needs of many individuals, provide cohesion and meaningful group commitment, and add to the rich fabric and complexity of world societies.

GENDER AND MENTAL HEALTH

Positive gender health is important to all people, including our teens and younger people. Gender health is how a person feels and presents themselves to the people close to them, their immediate contact groups, and the outside world. If a person identifies as non-binary, (they do not belong to either the male or female binary), and they may wish to dress in a way that feels appropriate to them and their personality; if this is so, they should be allowed to do so without prejudice from other people!

To qualify, gender is how a person feels inwardly, how they see themselves from the 'inside out' and not the 'outside in!' For instance, a male or female may see themselves as non-binary, but either male or female may present an image to the world if they are a male from birth, (their natal sex), but present to the world as a female!

BISEXUALITY

Bisexuality is a general identity used or given to those people who mix with and have sex with both males and females!

PHYSICAL EXPRESSION AND APPEAL

The Ancient Greeks loved the physical form of the human body! We only need to look at the Greek Goddess, Artemis, to see how the female form was admired. We see presented the breasts of the female but exposure to the genitals is discretely covered with fine flowing fabric. Still today, we marvel at the natural shapes of fit athletes, in both the male and female form. It is this inherent admiration for the human being that drives, not only many commercial industries but our desires to see and want more of what we are seeing...!

EMOTIONS – BOTH NEGATIVE AND POSITIVE

It is the emotional reaction in response to either an event or visual image that stimulates your emotional response. For instance, when you see or experience something that pleases you, you feel the joy of the experience, if you experience something that hurts you, you feel sad, maybe angry, and other associated emotions which may include frustration...!

Your physical expression may be related to past experiences and memories of different experiences.

AROUSAL

When you see a person that leaves an impression on your memory and you cannot stop thinking about them, you not only have the stirring of emotions, but you have a chemical reaction within the hormones within your body and brain. The pleasure hormone is oxytocin! This hormone is an arousal state hormone that triggers sexual desires and the feeling of possibly mating or being closer and enjoying that person on a deeper level.

If you see a person and you are aroused, and that person is in another relationship, it may cause you problems. Also, not all arousal states are reciprocated!

When you become aware of your own internal and emotional state, it allows you to become mindful of how your mind and body respond to different people you meet in everyday life.

If the oxytocin levels of two people meeting are mutually high, the body will send out messages through clever body language to the other person or receiver. Some of the responses that the receiver may witness are fully dilated eye pupils, colouring of the lips may change to a deeper pink or red! The stance and body movement of the signaller will also change, the feet will become wider apart indicating that sexual interaction is available, and the signaller's body may lean forward to be closer to the other person!

All such signals can be sent without a word being spoken, a message being written down, or a text message sent...!

When signals are received and accepted, the sender of the message may go to the next move, which would be to touch! The touch may only be slight in the first instance! If the response from the receiver is positive, the receiver will send a subtle message back either through moving closer, through interconnected eye contact, smiling or through some other acceptance signal that will allow more actions to be taken.

All the reactions spoken about on the previous page are inherent and within a person, and each of us is within our personalities. Sex, after all, is the primary driver for the survival of the human species!

By understanding your emotions, you become alert and mindful which allows you to make informed decisions and respond effectively to different situations.

Though, we might receive many of the above signals in our daily interactions with other people, it is the boundaries we set ourselves that keep us safe and work to keep the world societies together.

If human beings followed their instincts and did not have boundaries, there would be many divorces and a lot of pain for individuals and families, and as responsible adults, when a commitment is entered into, there are rules to be obeyed!

BODY IMAGE INCLUDES BODY SHAPE, AND PHYSICAL MAKEUP ALSO INCLUDING HAIR COLOUR, EYE COLOUR, NOSE SHAPE, SKIN COLOUR, AND HEIGHT

Within the heading, of Physical Expression and Appeal, many of the topics below have come into the conversation. The following headings also have a direct impact on your visual senses and will trigger emotional responses from you.

- ✓ Body image.
- ✓ Body shape.
- ✓ Physical makeup, hair, and eye colour.
- ✓ Nose shape.
- ✓ Skin colour.
- ✓ Height.

And the list goes on!

Many different attributes or assets make each person appealing to another person! All and more of the signals spoken of in the above relate to the chemical reaction in you, when you experience and meet a person that triggers an emotional reaction or response!

SOCIALISATION

What is socialisation? Adults adapt their socialisation skills when they find they are in a new situation or entering a new relationship. When you enter a new relationship, there may be different norms and customs that need to be learnt. Socialisation teaches people what is expected of them in particular situations and different environments within the relationship!

When you or we enter different relationships, though the guidelines may be unspoken, there are norms of control that need to be understood. Socialisation may have cultural expectations, gender or role model guidelines and accepted or expected behaviours that are part of the structure of the relationship.

At the onset of any new relationship, tread carefully, because there is a lot of learning to do. Some of the learning may not meet your expectations, if this happens, speak about your experiences, and ask if 'modifications' can be made.

For effective socialisation to take place, honesty will need to be part of the conversation. Of course, if the new relationship is for a short time, the socialisation undertaken maybe with a view of 'working for a short time only...!' If this is so, many minor adjustments can be made to keep the relationship working while there is a possible end date in view.

If entering a relationship for a short period, but the end date is extended and extended, a more structured approach may be needed! By doing this, both partners will have a direction and a goal to work toward.

Using the pyramid opposite, and after reading this last chapter, review your situation and fill in the blank spaces as you now see yourself. Your views may change by the time you finish the book.

How To Create a Sexual and Loving Relationship

ARE YOU SEEING LIFE CHANGES DIFFERENTLY?

Sometimes, we need to change and modify our behaviours and indeed, the way we have previously thought about different things or behaviours. Modification can be done, but all relationships need to be in balance and on equal ground!

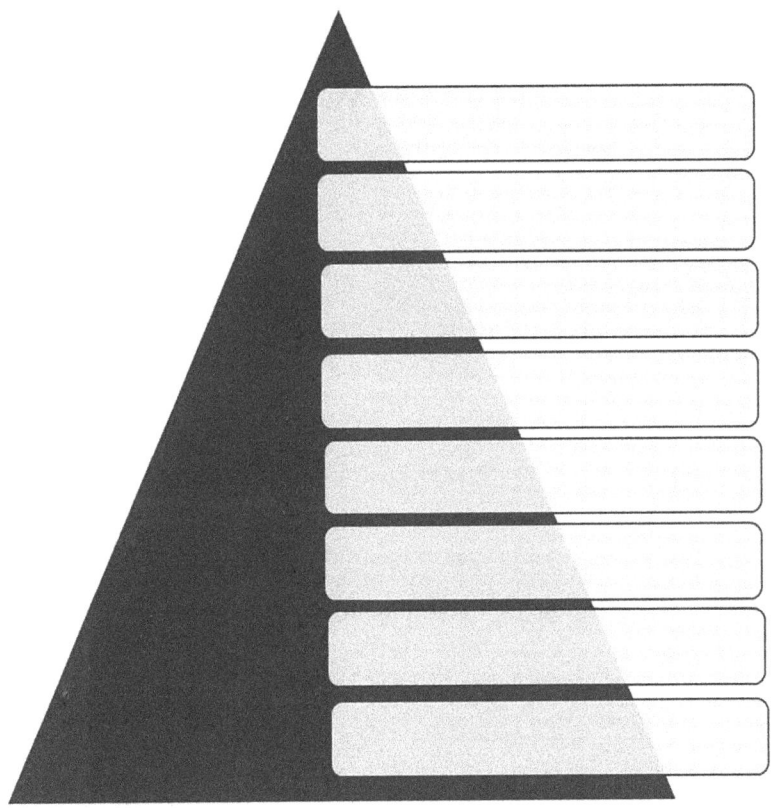

Copyright C Thompson-Wells 2024 ©

YOUR THOUGHTS

How To Create a Sexual and Loving Relationship

The 'How?' & 'Why?' of Hormones

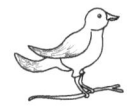 

CHAPTER FOUR
Fascination hormones...!

The ground was laid, I had taught sex education for three years and the children were bored with the subject. Some even said, 'Not again, miss, I did this last year!' I knew the children had greater capacities for learning than the simple, ineffective information I was given to teach!

As time went on and listening to the frustrations of the children, I knew something was missing in what they were being taught, simply, there wasn't a 'HOW?' and 'WHY?' within the information they were given, and the learning they were trying to do! Every piece of information given out to either children or adults should have a purpose with positive outcomes for the learner, this was not being achieved by the material given to teach...!

It is the lack of 'HOW?' and 'WHY?' in most information we read on how relationships, and other areas of human interest and fascination work, or don't work, that leads me to write so many of the books I write! In all human relationships, there are chemical interactions, some of the reactions we see, but many we don't...!

The human body and indeed the human brain is an intricate combination of human technology that has taken about six million years to develop and modify! As humans, we can identify as homo sapiens and have been walking the earth as this species for roughly, and as previously said, the last three to four hundred thousand years. We have come into existence through many generations of ancestors, all of which have contributed to refining and modifying our bodies, brains, and cell structures through each successful generation! Of course, those modifications to our physiology, and biology, including the cell structure, and the parts that help us to live our daily lives, may not be seen for generations. As each generation comes into being, it brings with it, its own body, brain, and cell modifications!

It is the advancement of technology that enables us to have the knowledge we have and indeed the knowledge that supports me in writing the books I write.

It is with fascination that I watch Professor Brian Cox as he gives us valuable knowledge and allows us to understand, not only how the universe came into being, but how we too have developed through many millions of years.

It is the way that many cells work in your body that allows you to see and feel the chemical reactions when a possible partner enters your life.

In the previous chapter, I mentioned oxytocin, which is but one chemical that works within your system when you register a liking for another human being!

Not all relationships are sexual, though at first, that may have been the immediate intention, some relationships may start with sexual thoughts and desires, but they may move into being long and beautiful friendships...

LET'S TALK ABOUT HORMONES
Without hormones working in your body and brain, you would possibly walk this earth as a type of living robot! You may meet up with a similar member of your species

How To Create a Sexual and Loving Relationship

to have sex and make babies, but there would be none of the passion that makes sex and relationships interesting or exciting! Hormones allow us humans to have this fascination in our lives. Hormones allow us to feel happy, sad, cautious, angry, frightened, and to fall in love!

Human fascination is what makes the world we live in, the place it is today and as we know, there has been this fascination for thousands of years!

Hormones, as in the human sex hormones, of which, many have a 'use by date!' Following, I have used some of my teens' puberty book images to illustrate how hormones work in the human body and brain, alongside the Hormones with Hats images and the chemical constructs.

The images are comical, but the message they deliver within your body's system and brain is far from comical.

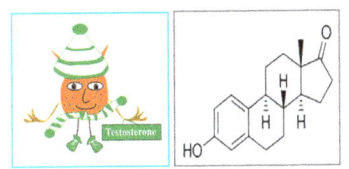

TESTOSTERONE

When young boys develop during puberty, it is

testosterone that supports the boy to become an adult male. It is at this point, boys will start to experience penis erections and wet dreams, (the natural release or ejaculation of sperm while the boy or young adult sleeps.) The release of sperm shows the penis is working and in good form and is doing what is meant to be done! The release of sperm, which may be old sperm, makes way for new sperm and is helping to keep the penis healthy and functional.

Both males and females have testosterone in their bodies. For females, testosterone may be in lower quantities than in males! Testosterone helps to balance the female hormones and helps with the female menstrual cycle balance.

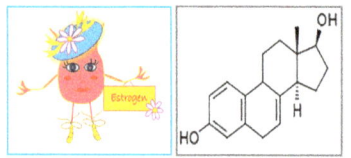

ESTROGEN

The hormone story is big, bold, and interesting! So, when a female develops into womanhood, she has a greater flow of estrogen and other womanly hormones which help each female as she develops.

Estrogen is the name given to a group of hormone compounds. It is a main hormone and is essential to the menstrual cycle which can go from twenty-one to thirty-five days. Estrogen helps the body to mature. It also helps to make the female's bones stronger and to keep the heart and brain healthy.

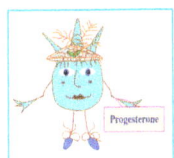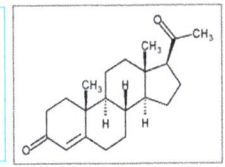

PROGESTERONE

Progesterone is a hormone produced and released from the female ovaries. It helps when females start to have their periods and help in the body's control of the menstrual cycle.

Before fertilisation, it supports the function of human sperm in the migration through the female vaginal tract after intercourse. Progesterone plays a key role in breast development and supports the maturation of breasts (mammary glands) during pregnancy which allows for lactation to develop allowing the mother to breastfeed her infant.

Studies have shown that progesterone supports normal neuron and brain development, and if damaged, the hormone has a protective effect on brain-damaged tissue.

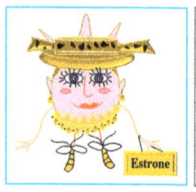 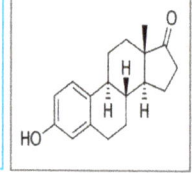

ESTRONE

Estrone can store estrogen and helps with female development and plays a part in female reproductive health. Like many hormones, estrone works with the female body clock. Many hormones can be sensitive to any body changes.

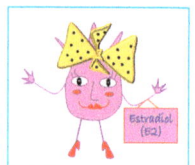 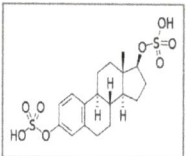

ESTRADIOL

Estradiol is also a female hormone produced primarily in the female ovaries. Estradiol levels can vary depending on the phase of the female menstrual cycle. Males also produce estradiol in their bodies. Estradiol levels can vary depending on the phase of the female menstrual cycle. It is also involved with the adjustment of the female reproductive cycle. During puberty it supports the development of breasts, the widening of the hips, and the fat distribution within the body. It also helps the female body in the maintenance of the reproductive tissue within the uterus and the breasts.

Its positive contribution also helps with maintaining healthy body tissue, bone, fat, skin, liver, and the human brain.

ESTRIOL

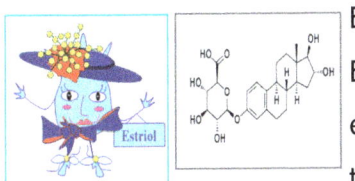

Estriol, like estrone, and estradiol, helps the female body to grow and become ready for womanhood. Like so many hormones, it too, works with its clock and will click into gear when it receives certain messages from the brain.

We are each far more complicated within our chemistry and human construction than just the feelings and desires that go with individual human emotions. When our emotions kick in, so do our hormones and a host of other chemicals that allow us to think and behave like human beings!

Having outlined the hormones in the illustrations seen on the previous pages is by no means a minimisation of the work they do! The hormone oxytocin, as so many people know is the 'love' hormone, but levels of oxytocin are known to vary...!

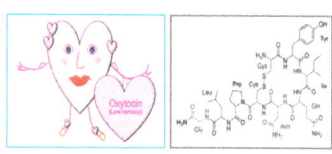

OXYTOCIN
This hormone is particularly interesting because, research from trusted sources, is telling us that low oxytocin levels may contribute to sadness, depression, and other negative feelings. Having said that, when your oxytocin levels are responsive to other people and your heart misses a beat on seeing a person, maybe for the first time, you know your oxytocin levels are working and in good form!

HORMONES NEED TO BE TRIGGERED
Your hormones work within your endocrine system, hormones are indeed, chemical messengers that carry information around your body, and to and from your brain. For instance, you have the ghrelin hormone within

the stomach and this hormone lets you know when you are hungry. The message from your stomach runs up your spine through what is known as the brain/gut neuron axis. It is the message received from the stomach that makes you think of food, and it is time to eat! This message to your brain can only be successful if the ghrelin hormone is successfully working!

Another thought, it is difficult to register and engage with your oxytocin if you are hungry and you need to have a food intake! This is where, going out and getting to know someone, is possibly better to do with a dinner date...!

YOUR SENSES AND THEIR ROLE IN MEETING OTHER PEOPLE

Collecting information for the books has taken many years and in working in many different environments. Possibly, the most powerful of teaching environments is with young, inquisitive students, who just want more and more information; they become like sponges asking the 'How?' and 'Why?' questions and that type of response triggers my yearning to find out the answers to give the information back to the students!

It is this 'How?' and 'Why?' that pushes on in most of us and leads us to explore and learn. We have discussed only some of your body's hormones, but it is the senses that trigger the hormones that make us ask vital questions and seek the necessary answers!

When you first see or meet a new possible partner, it is either through your visual acceptance, or if you hear somebody on the phone, it is through the sound of their voice. Both seeing and hearing incorporate your visual and hearing senses. The message is received into your brain where you start accumulating the information about this person.

Your senses work in conjunction with your brain which incorporates an electrical feedback loop of data. Now, please remember, it is not only the visual and hearing senses that are working but also your hormone supply. You may see aspects of this person's personality that don't sit comfortably with you, but you may sexually desire them, this is the oxytocin and other sex hormones that may override your common sense. The human desire to mate can be at times, powerful, and many people may find having sex difficult to resist! Remembering, from scientific research, '...*we are hard-wired to want and have sex...!*'

If both people are of legal age and have consented to the act, keeping in mind that consent is part of respect for each other and each other's body, some short interactions are accepted by both people. However, if the act of making love happens while an individual is already in another, established relationship, the act, may cause pain and hurt within that relationship! With all matters considered, it then becomes an individual choice.

YOUR SENSES CONTINUED
Your senses are connected to your nervous system and run throughout every part of your body. The nervous system is on both the inside of your body and close to your skin's surface! This is why touching the skin of

another person can be seen as an accepted behaviour or a violation! All aspects of behaviour should be understood before advances are made. Though I can sit and write this information down, it can be very different in real-life situations!

SO, HOW DO YOUR SENSES WORK WITH YOUR BRAIN? Your human body and brain are beyond marvellous, they are indeed advanced technology that is way ahead of any computer built to date. Your nervous system works in two ways, 1) your gross motor which allows you to move away from someone, run, jump, and other physical motor movements, and 2) your sensory systems allow you to feel touch, hot, cold, and other sensory experiences, including making love, the passion of the moments and the feeling of closeness to another person.

The core of your nervous system lies within the composition of your brain and spinal cord; the spinal cord carries your Central Nervous System (CNS) which allows all parts of your body to be connected to your brain.

Your nervous system is a naturally organised structure of cells and nerve endings that run throughout your body and brain. Within your brain, you have a 'response centre' that works with your body and triggers responses to stimuli such as touch, cold, hot, pain, sweetness, sour, and others, and this is why, when you are touched by another person, you can immediately register the 'touch!'

Your brain also has a separate but interconnected nervous system which contains the 'nerve centre' which works with the olfactory nerves for sight and smell. Your brain is a busy place as your nervous systems receive input from the spinal cord and the Peripheral Nervous Systems (PNS).

The PNS is a collection of organic ganglia[4] that sends messages to and from your brain which gives messages to incoming stimuli. The PNS is close to the surface of your skin, this is why, if cutting fruit or vegetables ready

---

[4] Groups of tissue containing neuron cell bodies that can categorised as either sensory or autonomic.

for a meal and you cut into the skin of your finger, it can sting or feel painful!

So, when you are 'touched,' it is your brain allowing you to make decisions within the 'nerve centre,' of your brain, that alerts and directs you to make the next behaviour happen. With 'touch,' you may move or move away or accept the advancement!

It is your senses working with the nervous system that allows you to respond to different life situations and your environment.

Most of us have heard the term, 'eye candy!' Much sugared candy is bad for the human body, and equally so, some 'eye candy' can be visually appealing but lack in substance and worth. It may be the instant attractiveness of another person that appeals to a person and holds their attention to explore and investigate more of what they are seeing! When 'eye candy' seems to be better in the packaging than the substance within, then it is time to move out and remove yourself from the attractiveness, regardless of what your eyes are telling you. Our senses can override our common sense at times and many people have been caught up in situations they wish they had never entered!

You will be familiar with the six areas of your body that work within your sensory system:

1. For visual, your eyes
2. For hearing, your ears
3. For touch, your skin
4. For smell, your nose
5. For taste, your tongue, and the senses of taste and
6. For balance, your body needs to regulate how you move and navigate different terrains such as sitting, standing, walking, running or in travel!

REACTIONS TO 'EYE CANDY!'
FIRST STEPS – YOUR HUMAN BODY AND BRAIN
The human body contains over one billion neurons that are within the spinal cord and brain. There are twelve pairs of nerves directly linked to the brain. These nerves

are called cranial nerves that help to support your heart rate, movement, senses, and other sensory stimulations. This is why, when seeing a person that stimulates your arousal, you may feel your heart miss a beat, you may feel sweating, or your pupils may dilate; all such bodily reactions are stimulated by the visual image and the messages sent to your brain for analysis.

The first perceptual image may be an illusion, or not in reality to the real person. Many relationships are entered into through the perception of an image, but the person does not turn out to be the image first seen....!

In some instances, we may want a person in our lives but what we may see as 'eye candy' in the first instance, may contain the remnants of your past relationships, and experiences, a mixture of culture, some hidden desires, and the willingness to have an attachment to someone else!

Meeting new people is always a nervous time in life, most of us have reservations, and some move into relationships with caution, but sometimes we may 'throw caution to the wind,' and suffer the consequences...!

If you feel this is identifying you or parts of you, please take some time out to think about and re-adjust to your current situation.

Of course, some people meet and instantly there is a match; the chemistry is right and each fits the other person's values. If adjustments are needed, they are accommodated and done with consideration and over time.

YOUR EYES AND VISUAL INSIGHT

Your occipital lobe, which lies towards the back of your brain, please see the image, works with the images you see. The processing of the image, as in 'eye candy,' is done through the information within your temporal lobe; this is the lobe at the side of your head. You can gently touch your temple and

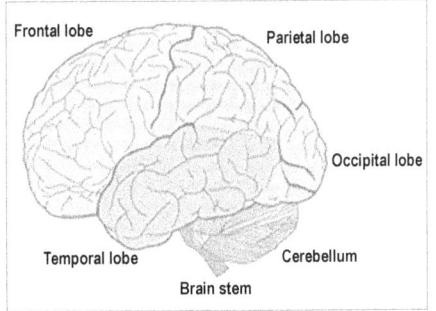

Image, Courtesy Wiki Commons

directly within your head, your temporal lobe sits at the side of your skull. This lobe helps you to analyse and process the visual images you see from your occipital lobe. If in the vision of the 'eye candy,' you see a resemblance to a past love, it is the remnants, and memory held within the temporal lobe that is stimulated!

Please remember, you cannot replace people; each person is unique and a separate individual.

HEARING THE VOICE

A person that has a character voice or a distinctive voice is difficult to not want 'more of the sound' of the voice! Again, the temporal lobe has stored the information of voices you may like or the voice of somebody you don't want to hear!

Your temporal lobe is responsible for processing sound, which is done through the auditory complex within the temporal lobe.

YOUR NOSE – ITS SENSITIVITY

Your nose has highly charged nerve endings. The sense of smell is the oldest of your senses and is associated with the olfactory bulb at the back of your nose.

Well, you may ask, what has this got to do with sex, sexuality, and relationships? Your sense of smell is connected to your brain and memories, the smell of another person may contribute or reduce your liking of that person!

Past civilisations have long been aware of perfumes and have known that our bodies have different odours which has inspired the development of different perfumes and creams. In some instances, perfumes and creams have been developed to cover bad odours, however, in other instances, perfumes have been used as sexual enticement tools to attract other people to us...!

The use of body perfumes dates to about four thousand years ago. The oldest use of perfume may have been in the burning of incense and other aromatic gums and herbs, all of which are still very much used today. Perfumes enhance the ambience for seduction, lovemaking, and the preparation of the mind to enjoy the moments that follow.

Perfumes play other roles,

- Can reduce body odour.
- Be used as an aphrodisiac.
- Change and enhance moods.
- Add comfort and be soothing to the brain when inhaled.
- Add to confidence and be intoxicating in certain environments and atmospheres.
- Allow for stillness within the environment so that special moments become lifelong good memories.
- Add to the attractiveness of the moments and the intimacy of the time.

So, given the above, it makes sense to try out the recipe, but please, only enjoy the moments when you are safe and with a person you trust.

With a word of caution, your sense of smell will also warn you and will,

- Trigger memories, both good and bad.

We have spoken about 'eye candy,' a derogatory description to many, but it fits with the times we are currently living in and within many general conversations going on around the world.

So, how does this all work?

HOW YOUR BODY & BRAIN SYSTEMS WORK

1) Messages from your environment are picked up by your senses.
2) The messages are transmitted through your nervous system to your brain.
3) Your brain explores the information from the thoughts and information you have.
4) From the analysis, you make choices.
5) From the choice, you act in either the words you speak or the movement/actions you take!
6) Then there are outcomes from your actions you've made or taken…!

Now that you have finished Chapter Four, please take some time to review your feelings and change or modify the very good assets that belong to you.

As you go through the chapters, you are building on your emotional intelligence by the information you are gathering and will use now and into your future.

ARE YOU SEEING DIFFERENCES IN THE WAY YOU THINK AND FEEL?

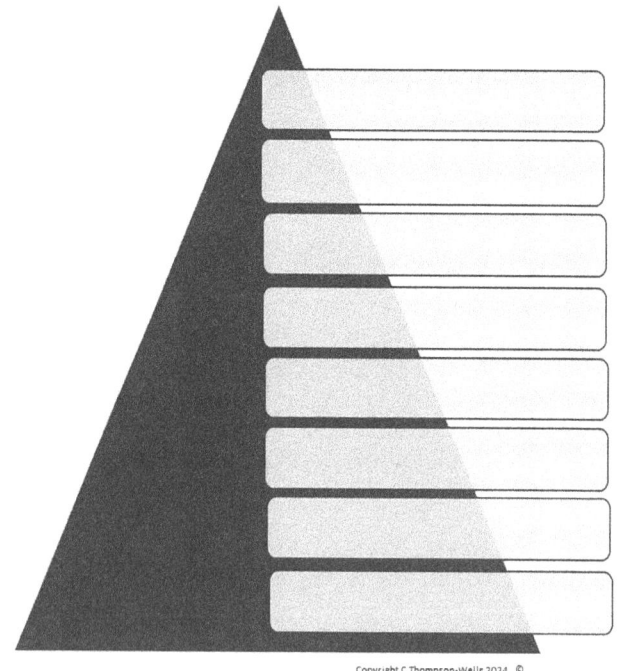

YOUR THOUGHTS

How To Create a Sexual and Loving Relationship

Sex Hormones – Their Working Capacity...

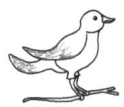 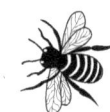

CHAPTER FIVE
Let's talk about sex hormones!

When we are children, we may often think about when we grow up, at that time, we may go through many imagined scenarios, and say, 'When I grow up...!' During this period of realisation, we have no idea and little knowledge as to the complexity of life and of human behaviours and relationships!

Children should be allowed to be children, but if we want our children to grow up with the knowledge of how loving, healthy relationships work, and what is needed to keep treasured relationships together, we need to understand, as adults, how our human emotions work, and how they play a vital part in the relationships we have!

Having taught and been in the classroom teaching the subjects of psychology, sex or puberty, and other life skill education, it is still in disbelief, that I look at my childhood and see how little I knew or was told about sex and relationships. It is possibly, a sign of the times, but many people still cannot face the reality of the times we are living in and the exposure we all must, sometimes, see, the aggressive social media and the images that are plunged in front of us on the phone and other screens!

YOUR NOSE AND INTIMACY
We've already spoken about your senses and your body's electrical systems, but now, we will go a little deeper and speak about how the smell sense is triggered or the role it plays in relationships!

For your nose to register smell, it must receive the scent from the air via inhaling through your nose. The essence of the smell or perfume is carried in small molecules[5] through the air and on hitting your nose, the molecule is transported, through the breathing you are doing, to your brain. The information journey of the molecule is far more complicated than what is written here, but if

---

[5] A molecule is made up of a glycerol head with three fatty acid tails each of which is a hydrogen and carbon chain. Molecules are so small; they cannot be seen with the naked eye. They are in the air you breathe, the water you drink and the food you eat. ©

you imagine an electrical system, which is what the neuron pathways of our brains and bodies provide. You will understand that every essence of the perfume of the microscopic molecule must go on its electrical journey which at the end of the journey is the smell your brain registers! You either like, love, or dislike the molecule smell you are receiving…! If the relationship is to continue, you will accept the aromas, smells, or perfume; if you find the molecules upsetting, you will either continue with the activity or find an excuse to hastily retreat…!

Your association with incoming smells is primeval and handed down by your ancestors. Your smell sense has allowed you to keep safe, for instance, you will be alarmed, through the smell of fire and if the fire is close to you; you will look at ways to escape to save your life! Your nose lets you know if the food you are about to eat is good for eating or on the turn…! Your sense of smell also plays a role in how you perceive the incoming smell of another person, this is all part of any relationship which needs to be understood[6].

If the information from the molecule is delightful and you are responding to the natural smell or the essence of the perfume, your hormones will interact with your brain's electrical system, and you will start to feel the pleasure of the experience.

Relationships and building relationships are about your senses, the positive interaction of your hormones, and the emotions you experience!

All people, regardless of cleanliness, have their own unique odour and it is this odour you will enjoy or dislike. This is all part of the chemistry of people and relationships!

---

[6] Most normal body smells or odours are natural. Your nose is sensitive and will send alarms to your brain if the odours change or are different!

YOUR SKIN AND INTIMACY

Most people love to have their skin touched. How many people, even within strong relationships, like to have a massage, and so many thousands around the world daily have this pleasure?

From trusted sources, our research shows that people who have regular massage, especially those who live alone or in singular accommodation, such as university students and others studying, or those living away from home, older people living in homes or care centres and others; a massage can add an extended quality to their life. It is the gentle touch of the skin that relaxes the nervous system and in turn, those feel-good hormones such as:

- Dopamine
- Serotonin
- Oxytocin
- Endorphins

Are released into the body and supported by the brain and the brain's functions that allow the positive flow of chemicals to flow easily through the body, relaxing the muscles and other areas of the torso, limbs, and head.

These hormones are connected to the Pleasure Centre which sits within the brain of both males and females!

Now let's identify how these hormones will add benefits to you and your relationship!

DOPAMINE

Dopamine is the 'feel good' hormone, dopamine is a neurotransmitter[7], and functions as part of your brain's reward system. Dopamine loves a party, pleasurable experiences, sensations, and excitement. Dopamine functions allow you to learn new skills, and new life experiences and support both good and not-so-good memories. There is a downside to dopamine, when your natural supply of dopamine is low, you can feel sad, have mood swings, feel irritable, and have bouts of

---

[7] As a teacher of psychology, I understand that a neurotransmitter carries chemical messengers, such as dopamine, which facilitates communication between neurons in the brain and nervous system.

depression, which can leave you feeling exhausted and lacking in energy...!

A way to naturally increase dopamine levels is to do something you enjoy and do it the minute you realise that you are feeling sad or depressed. Even smiling at yourself in the mirror and seeing your reflection can bring a natural smile to your face. This one action will alert your dopamine supply and the natural supply will increase...

Because dopamine is the 'feel good' hormone and if there is an oversupply, like too much adrenaline, it may lead you into dangerous situations, always think from the 'inside out' and do not be tempted by what is offered to you from the outside...! Meaning, be cautious if you are in 'party mode,' and want more of what may not be good for you...!

SEROTONIN
Relationships and the connections to other people you have in different relationships can play on your mind and

this is possibly more so when you go to bed and want to sleep!

Serotonin is known as the natural sleep hormone, but sometimes, serotonin is in short supply when sleep is wanted!

Stress, worries and other daily concerns can interfere with your serotonin levels! If this happens, you may lose interest in learning, your memory and recall of different situations may be hampered, your digestive system may cause you concern, you may have interrupted sleep, and sleeping problems, and you may lose some of your sex drive…!

Serotonin is an important hormone for both mind, brain and body wellbeing. Prior, to going to bed, doing relaxation exercises, doing a hobby which you enjoy, regular breathing exercises, and having some 'ME' time can all assist in raising your serotonin levels. Now, and in some countries, natural serotonin products may be bought over the counter! You may wish to seek medical advice if you think your serotonin levels are low or if this is a health concern!

On the upside of serotonin, it is a neurotransmitter that helps regulate your mood, appetite, digestion, and memory and adds to your quality of life and sleep, it also adds to your interest in pleasurable behaviours, including your love life...!

OXYTOCIN

The hormone oxytocin is also a chemical messenger that is produced by the hypothalamus in your brain but is stored in the pituitary gland. It plays many roles in human behaviour including human interaction, and sexual arousal, it helps to promote bonding in relationships and empathy which promotes physical affection, love and tenderness. Oxytocin helps the womb to contract in labour, it supports uterine contractions during childbirth and in lactation for the newborn after birth.

For males, oxytocin helps in the production of testosterone and the movement of sperm.

On the downside, low levels of oxytocin are seen when there is an inability to feel and show affection, there is difficulty in reaching an orgasm, and there are increased levels of anxiety and disturbed sleep.

As with so many of the 'feel good' hormones, oxytocin levels can be increased naturally through doing the things or hobbies you love to do, for example, gentle exercising or meditation, listening to your type of music, something that will soothe, rather than 'head banging...', having a massage, having a cuddle or hug, and patting your pets.

Oxytocin helps in sexual arousal, sexual enjoyment and the satisfaction of the moments during the act of sex.

ENDORPHINS
Like the previously spoken about hormones, endorphins are chemical messengers and are produced in your

pituitary gland and hypothalamus, both located in your brain. Endorphins are released when you feel stress or pain or if you feel, you are in a difficult situation and are looking for a solution. Endorphins, through their ability to reduce stress, allow you to think more clearly, and improve your mood. It is this ability that makes you a survivor.

Your endorphin levels can be boosted through exercising, eating a healthy diet, having a massage, doing the things you enjoy doing, and having sex!

By understanding how your 'feel good' hormones work, you will greatly improve your health and well-being, allow you to work constructively from the 'inside out' and stay on top of many situations you may encounter daily.

Hormones, emotions, and your body's electrical system all play their part in how you live your life. It is the interconnection of hormones, emotions, and your body's electrical systems, together with your senses of seeing and touching that trigger your reactions within your relationships.

FEMALE AND MALE SEX HORMONES

FEMALES: 1) Progesterone, 2) Estrogen, 3) Estrone, 4) Estradiol and 5) Estriol.

MALES: 1) Testosterone, 2) Androgens, and 3) Inhibin.

It is the drive of the above hormones, together with your emotions that allows love and sex to take place.

It may be time to rethink! Having read the information so far, have your values and assets changed?

OBSESSION AND INFATUATION

It is when you or we meet somebody, who exudes sex appeal, and the feeling overpowers you, it goes beyond physical attraction, it may be a love journey or become an obsession or infatuation; these mental states can become a fixation and be fascinating; these relationships can also be dangerous!

If through your observations during a relationship, you have any warning from your subconscious mind, you should heed the warnings! In dangerous obsession, it is the human mind that contains the power of thought, thinking (cognition), analysis, deduction, and judgment.[8] When taken notice, the power of your mind gives you warnings or can equally enjoy the moments of a re-vitalising relationship.

YOUR NOTES

....

....

....

....

....

....

....

....

....

....

---

[8] C Thompson-Wells, (2016) 'Stop Family Violence Now.'

YOUR THOUGHTS AND VALUES – HAVE THEY CHANGED?

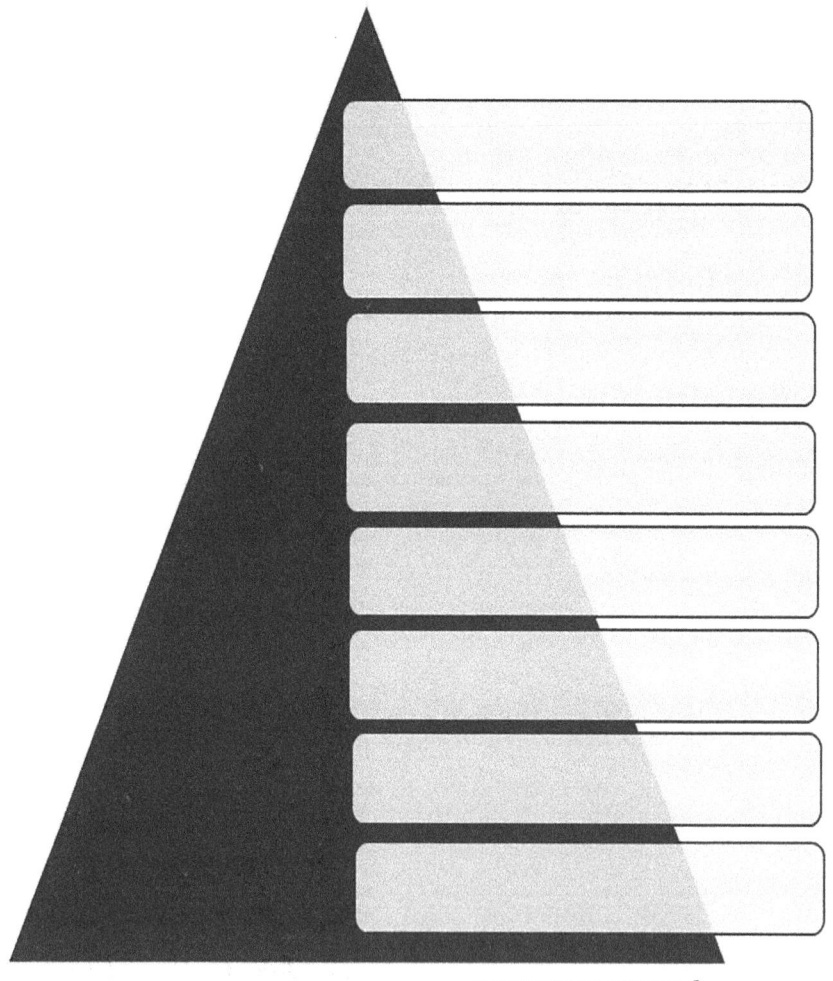

YOUR NOTES

How To Create a Sexual and Loving Relationship

The Human Body...

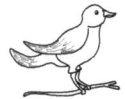 

CHAPTER SIX
Understanding sex: the male and female body

It has been a bit of a journey to brace myself and to write a book that speaks openly about our human sexual behaviour, but, at this point, I have only covered part of the story, there is still more to come!

To begin this chapter, and to mention again, for many thousands of years, there has been a fascination with the human body and how it works! In Chapter One, I discussed the many male images of phallus, seen throughout history, through many cultures, in different parts of the world, and through recorded human history. Not only were there images of the male genitals, but the female genitals are seen in some cultural antiquities. And here we are in the Twenty-First Century and still the fascination continues!

THE MALE – FROM A BOY TO A MAN
The penis grows and matures as the male child develops and goes into puberty. The testes and the scrotum

develop with the scrotum becoming larger as the testes start to produce sperm; this is all a natural part for the male when growing up...!

The following illustrations are taken from my children's and teens' puberty books.

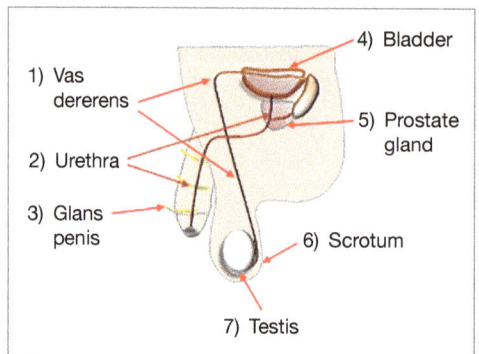

I am writing for adults here and without repeating myself, the illustrations are self-explanatory and can be followed.

In the next illustration, it shows how the sperm travels through the penis and urethra network until the sperm is released at the time of ejaculation.

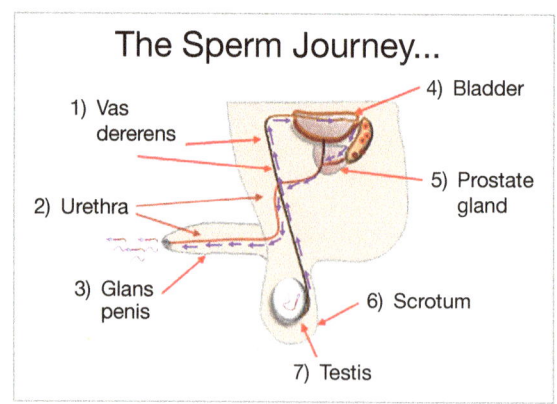

Sperm leaves the penis at a speed of about forty-five kilometres, or faster, an hour! This is always funny to the listener, or reader, but it is a fact! The reason sperm travels so fast is, during lovemaking and intercourse, the sperm's goal is to fertilise the female egg and for such a tiny cell, (which is the smallest cell in the human body), it takes energy! Energy, in the form of starches, proteins, and hormones, and on the journey out of the male, the energy is provided by the prostate gland.

In a healthy male, the testes will continue to produce sperm until he dies. Making sperm by the testes is an ongoing process with a healthy male making up to one million, nine hundred thousand sperm each day! Each month, the female produces, on average, one egg! Unlike females, males do not go through menopause as in the female sense, but a male, as he becomes older, may produce less sperm because of the decline in the manufacturing of testosterone produced in his testes. If this is so, the male's inclination to have sex or intercourse may reduce or stop!

Remedies, solutions, or medical advice are not a part of this book's contents, but if you have concerns, please seek professional medical advice and instruction.

Let's move on, there are no statistics given to show how many times the sexual act is acted on daily and around the world...! If we remove our children and younger people and those people over eighty years of age, it would possibly be close to, or a little less, than half of the world's population at any one time...!

If this is the case, why is the topic of the natural human body and how it works, such taboo in so many homes, community groups, and countries? We know from statistics showing, disaffected youth, more criminal gangs, human slavery, sex trafficking, and other violations of human beings, and in many instances, it is the lack of education that helps to promote crime and the abuse of people, sometimes caught up in the above situations.

The human body is a magnificent creation and having studied, and sculpted the human form, with live models while at university, the human form still, leaves me in wonderment!

When we commit to the sex act within any relationship, we are committing so with trust and understanding that we will be treated with respect and consideration. If any of the above: trust, understanding, respect, and consideration are not part of the union and relationship, then the time spent together will be agonising, and leave us wishing it would end sooner rather than later...!

THE SENSITIVITY OF THE HUMAN MOUTH

Few people realise, except for the medical profession, with the first kiss, there is the touching of the lips, a sensory sensation is sent to the brain, and then there is an exchange of human saliva from one person to another! If kissing doesn't happen when you make love, this next part of the information will not interest you...!

It is interesting, that humans have been kissing, (pashing) for thousands of years, we see it in films, and we go, 'Ah...' and little is thought about anything else other than romantic love! However, what is happening is again, a primeval act! The kissing promotes the exchange of saliva which contains, some mucus, proteins, salts, possibly starches, and enzymes. From our earlier times, kissing may have been an act of ownership and belonging, so if taken seriously, kissing may be a bonding activity!

The saliva of the mouth also plays other roles; it is released by glands that lubricate the mouth and aid in the digestion of food and the breaking down of food starches! In some acts of love, the mouth is used to caress the human body.

Once the kiss has passed the post of acceptance, the fondling begins. The fondling promotes sexual arousal from the messages received from your senses directly under your skin's surface, and from the visual and hearing messages received by your brain, at this point, or before, once stimulated, if you haven't already started, you may reciprocate the fondling...!

If it is all systems go, the female nipples will become firm, the male penis will already be erect, and the next move would be to go to the bedroom, find a room, or in some instances, find a convenient and safe place, and each other would remove parts or all their clothing!

A caution note, hasty sex, can be fraught with danger, and it is always wise to get to know the partner you are with, before committing to the sex act.

If we look at several happy movies, as in 'Love Actually,' the scene between Karl, (Rodrigo Junqueira Reis Santoro), and Sarah, (Laura Linney), film names, we can see and feel the agony of the moment, when Karl must come back to reality because of Sarah's constant incoming phone calls from her brother...!

It is during the intimate and special moments of our lives that we start to build memories of the experiences and the learning we are doing at that time!

SO, WHAT HAPPENS NEXT...?

Within healthy relationships, the penis is used as a means of connection, and togetherness. It allows for intimacy at one of the highest levels of human behaviour and is an act of love and admiration.

THE ERECTION OF THE PENIS

As the fondling and kissing continue, the ultimate moment comes when the couple is about to have their intimate moments.

For a penis to have an erection, there are many functions the body must perform. Each person within the act must be willing and accepting of what is going to happen next! When each person is comfortable with the situation, their brains are working, together with their bodies, and in unison to make the moments happen!

THE TISSUE AND MAKEUP OF THE MALE PENIS

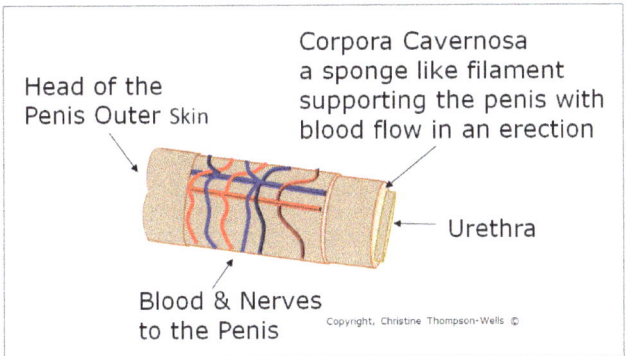

The above image displays, the head of the penis and the outer skin which shows the vein structure, just below the skin's surface. It also identifies the corpora cavernosa, a sponge-like tissue that fills with blood while in erection.[9] The female's body has a similar sponge-like tissue within the inner labium and folds, that, likewise, fills with blood during arousal and clitoral erection during sexual activities!

A male penis, through the interaction within the male's brain, can receive messages from different areas within his body. Like females, the male responds by using his senses.

---

[9] Image taken from my book, 'Hormones, Puberty & Your Child.'

As can be seen in the previous diagram, the penis is a complicated piece of human technology. It has an outer skin, a blood and nerve distribution network, and a sponge-like material, as mentioned above, that is made up of the corpora cavernosa. At the base of the penis is the urethra, which is the urine track that releases both urine and sperm.

It is the fondling and love play that excites both males and females during sex.

Just to mention here, sperm always takes priority over urine and will be released before urine. This is all part of the clever human body technology that has been working for thousands of years and through many generations of males in the world.

I have spoken about the body's nervous system which works through your body's electrical neuron pathways. During the act of sex, the nerves within the surface of the penis, within the surface of the walls of the female vagina, and the female clitoris, are nerve endings that are known as free nerves! And like all free things, they are always willing and ready to be touched, and are ready for the excitement, and pleasure that touch brings to the human body! It is during sex that these nerves operate to bring the maximum of pleasure to your lovemaking! Your nervous system is working with your free nerves which tell your brain of the pleasure you are experiencing!

Sex and lovemaking are serious human actions and behaviours and are meant to be enjoyed! For a female to become aroused she needs to have her body working and in good order.

Some sexual acts are done because they are part of a pre-existing contract, if this is the case, and if the togetherness is to continue, there may be some extra work to do! It takes dedication and possibly seeing each other in different ways, or making the intimate moments spent together, magical, and purposeful to fulfill many sexual desires and pleasures.

THE FEMALE BODY

The female body is equally as magnificent as the male body. As we all know, females have external breasts that can be of many different sizes and shapes! A female may be extremely proud of her breasts and why not, they are beautiful, and the curve of the female body is enhanced through both her bone shape within the hips, the shape of her breasts, and the vivaciousness of her figure!

Within the natal sex, the female body is constructed differently. Earlier, in the book, I spoke about chromosomes, when a female is born, she has, all the ingredients that make her into a sexual female later in life.

(To note, many males, females, and people have lived in partnerships for thousands of years and it is the chemistry of the mateship, regardless of a personally prescribed gender, that keeps couples and or groups together!)

THE FEMALE BODY CONTINUED

Because many of the sexual, female body parts are hidden and not easily seen, some females may feel embarrassed to speak about the vulva and clitoris. Let's now open that conversation.

Like males, and if you are a female, it is important for you to sexually explore your body; it is the exploration that leads you to the enjoyment of sexual activity. Enjoyment of your body is equally as important as the enjoyment of your eyes when you see something beautiful, and you just want to look and look again! Or when you hear something, and the sound is so magical, you just want more and more of the sound, and so it is with your body.

Not only is it important to explore your body for pleasure, but it is equally important to explore your body to check your health and well-being.

Within the sex of your body, explore how it feels to touch the clitoris and what movements or touch feel pleasurable for you! Once you know how and what is good for your clitoris, you will know that during sexual activity, some movements are pleasurable, while others may make you sore and uncomfortable!

It is this knowledge and the communication with your partner that will empower you and the enjoyment from the sexual activities you do and create!

THE MAKING OF A WOMAN'S BODY

When females are born, we know they are a girl because of the lack of the penis, and 'It's a girl!' But apart from the lack of a penis, the girl is born with complex and detailed body parts!

Taken again, from one of my children's puberty books is the simplified image of the female internal body workings we so often see.

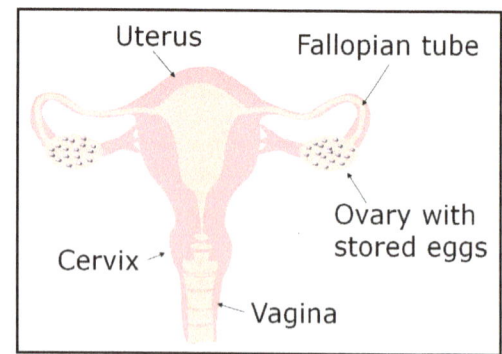

The female body is so much more complicated than this image, but it is at least a start for our children and teens!

Let's now go to other parts of the female body.

THE VULVA ALSO KNOWN AS THE PUDENDUM

The vulva, like the male penis, is sensitive to touch and when stroking or movement takes place, both the vulva and penis, through the many nerve endings and the body's neuron pathways, send messages to the human brain! These messages alert the brain to excitement, fascination, and pleasure…!

Once your brain is alerted to excitement, your pleasure-seeking hormones kick in, and as you now know, they are:

- ✓ Dopamine
- Serotonin
- Oxytocin
- Endorphins

As previously said, in the last chapter, 'these hormones are connected to the Pleasure Centre which sits within the brain of both males and females!' The pleasure centre loves any form of pleasure….!

A brief note here, for all readers, it is your brain's pleasure centre that can be overpowering and demanding, in the instance, you have tried drugs and to break the drug cycle, no drugs were to be taken, it is the withdrawal of the drug that your dopamine release becomes upset about!

Your brain has learnt, that releasing the hormone dopamine feels good, and more dopamine is released through the drugs being taken, soon, the recreational drug, that you thought was harmless at first, becomes so powerful, that it is almost impossible to resist taking more drugs!

In some instances, it is not only the release of dopamine but added to the concoction, maybe the hormone adrenaline!

Between your brain's pleasure centre, dopamine release from the hormone's gland and the effects of the drugs on your system, withdrawing from any bad habit may become difficult to do or achieve! When your brain's pleasure centre is overstimulated through developing a bad habit and that habit may be gambling, drinking too much alcohol, eating too much junk food or further habits that are not conducive to your good health and wellbeing, please think about your brain's pleasure centre! The brain's pleasure centre can become a dominant part of the personality, it can be demanding, and sometimes, demanding the almost impossible to be accomplished, but persistent you must be if you want to break a bad habit...!

A word about your brain, the brain is a very obedient servant, and if you give it a command, for instance, 'drink more wine...!' instead of 'don't drink more wine...!' The pleasure centre of your brain will encourage you to 'drink more wine...!' It is your responsibility and if you want to make positive changes in your life, to deny your pleasure centre's demands, and to be stronger than what the pleasure centre and the release of hormones are telling you to do...! Your pleasure centre can easily become your demand centre and bad habits are just that, they demand you to take an action, drug, including too much of anything that is not good for you! Once you take a stand, you may be breaking a bad habit that has dominated your life right up to this date, the choice is always yours...!

Let's now get back to the subject of sex and the female body!

It is the work of hormones that works through all sessions of sex, and sexual gratification.

The vulva is part of, but not unique to, the large bone at the front and lower part of the female trunk that, at puberty, grows and expands. The bone also known as the mons or mons pubis, forms the female mound shape that is part of the vulva. The vulva has a layer of fatty tissue that protects the bone and mound, and this helps to form the shape.

The shape or vulva seen on the outside of a woman's body forms an integral part of the female genital anatomy. This anatomy includes the mons, as previously spoken about, the pubis labia, which are the two folds of flesh which protect the female genital lower body openings, majora labia, and minora labia. The labia, during, the pregnancy of the mother, and in the development of the child, forms to protect the female genitals and are an essential part of the female's body's formation.

ANATOMY OF THE CLITORIS

The diagrammatic illustration following is just that, if you wish to find out more about the subject, please refer to trusted sources of medical research and information.

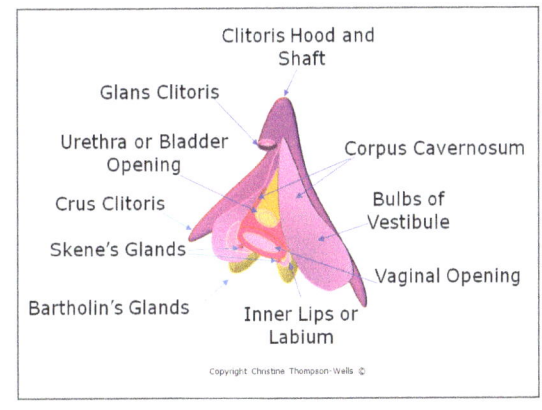

CLITORIS HOOD AND SHAFT

Please take a moment to study the previously seen illustration.

As can be seen in the opposite illustration, the female body parts are the clitoris, urethra, crus clitoris, Skene's glands, Bartholin's glands, inner lips or labium, vaginal opening, vestibular bulbs, and the corpus cavernosum.

The clitoris Glan is protected by the pubis labia, the outer soft tissue seen on the outside of the female body.

Each female is different, so many body shapes and parts can be different, but because of difference, it doesn't mean they are any less important, they are indeed, all very important!

And whilst bringing this information into the public arena, there still needs to be respect shown for the information given.

GLANS CLITORIS

The clitoris as already spoken about, is the pleasure centre of the female's reproductive anatomy. The clitoris consists of a complex network of erectile tissue and free nerve endings; some of these nerve endings are within the inner workings of the genitals, under the skin and close to the skin's surface.

Stimulating the clitoris can arouse sexual desires and allow a woman to become ready for lovemaking and romance. Stimulation heightens sexual tension until an orgasm happens. Having said that, not all females, though heightened sexually, will orgasm! Stimulation to the clitoris can make a female feel relaxed, loved, and cherished, it is indeed, a central connection within relationships.

There is much ongoing research at this time which shows that the clitoris is far more than a 'button' seen within the female vulva. The clitoris is a Glan, as is the penis, the male Glan. The female Glan, like the penis, and as previously said, contains 'free' nerve endings. According to recent research, *"It's starting to think about more than 10,000 nerve fibres being concentrated in something as small as a clitoris."*[10] Blair Peters. Indeed, there are more nerve endings in the clitoris than in any other part of the vulva!

The clitoris is extensive and has extended tissue inside the female body which runs along the wall of the vagina! There is no mystery about the clitoris, it is as much about the female body as the male penis is to the male body!

The entire clitoris from the glans to the crura is between three and a half inches to four and a half inches long (7.5-10cm) and about two and a half inches in diameter (6.5cm).

The body of the clitoris is located behind the Glans, which branches out, and surrounds the vaginal canal and urethra. The Crura has two leg shapes that extend from

---

[10] Blair Peters, a plastic surgeon at Oregon Health and Science University's School Medicine. We May Finally Know How Many Nerve Endings Are in The Human Clitoris. Article: HUMANS 05 November 2022 By CARLY CASSELLA

the clitoral body, these are 'V' shaped like an upside-down wishbone shape!

(To note, sexual arousal is any form of stimulation that enhances, sustains, and leads to an orgasm. In some instances, if you are a female and you are in good health, your body may naturally orgasm. This is a natural function of your body and is part of the body's maintenance system to keep your genital area healthy and functional. To naturally orgasm, is indeed a gift, and should be acknowledged and not taken for granted. A quiet 'thank you,' from you, acknowledging this gift is always a positive action sending good hormones throughout your body and brain!)

URETHRA OR BLADDER OPENING

The urethra or bladder opening in all natal sex females is close to the vaginal opening. Because of the structure and closeness of both orifices, females need to be ever vigilant about their hygiene in the genital areas of their bodies. Many women suffer from bladder infections, especially after intercourse. As my doctor once told me,

'Pee immediately, clean yourself down with, if available, a hygienic body wipe, and then dowse with clean flowing water...!' It works, but the action must be sooner, rather than later...!

(A note, it is not only females that need to keep their genital areas clean, but males also need to do so after intercourse. If you are a male, to clean, if a foreskin remains, gently pull the foreskin down and lightly clean, or if the foreskin has been removed as in circumcision, still consider the health of your body by taking care of the penis and clean accordingly.)

CRUS OR CRURA CLITORIS
Briefly mentioned under the heading Glans Clitoris, the crus clitoris is two erectile structures which form the 'V'-shape. Each leg of the 'V' is the corpus cavernosum on the clitoral body. Like the male penis, the corpus cavernosum has developed as a sponge-like tissue that fills with blood during clitoral erection.

SKENE'S GLANDS

The Skene's glands are not often spoken about in literature which include information on the female body, but they are an important working mechanism that helps natal sex females during intercourse! These glands are two small ducts located at either side of the urethra or bladder opening! They help to lubricate the vagina during sexual arousal and intercourse and contain certain protective mucus that helps with limiting infection. Some trusted research suggests that Skene's glands may be the source of orgasm or ejaculation in females.

Interestingly, the Skene's glands, in females, and from trusted sources, develop from the same cells as the prostate gland in natal males!

BARTHOLIN'S GLANDS

The Bartholin's glands are two pea-sized glands which contain ducts that function at the left and right of the vagina. Upon arousal, they also secrete a mucus that helps to lubricate the vagina. Again, like so many areas of the male and female genitalia, these are sensitive to touch or stimulation! The glands are paired and are open on the surface of the vulva.

INNER LIPS OR LABIUM

The labia are part of the function of the vulva which helps to protect the female sexual organs, urinary opening, vestibule, and vagina. The outer lips within the vulva are called the labia majora and the inner lips are known as the labia minora.

VAGINAL OPENING

Natal sex females start their periods at different times and through different ages. It is at the vaginal opening that a young female will experience her first sight of vaginal blood. Vaginal blood is not lifeblood. Vaginal blood is the blood that forms within the lining of the female uterus and at certain times of the month, this blood is naturally released forming the period.

In lovemaking between a male and female, it is the first penetration of the penis into the female vagina that forms the act of having sex. As said previously, if the act is between two consenting adults of legal age, the time spent together is for them to share and is a primeval part of the two natural bodies coming together to either enjoy each other or for the creation of another human being!

In many instances, it is the rubbing or touch of the penis within the walls of the vagina that allows a female to orgasm!

Research is ongoing as to the relationship between the clitoris and the Grafenberg spot or 'G' spot which it is commonly called. The 'G' spot is located a few inches within the vaginal opening; this may feel especially pleasurable or exciting when stimulated.

Both the male and female genital areas are known as erogenous[11] zones. People are different, and what excites some people, may not excite another!

---

[11] An erogenous zone of the human body that is sensitive to touch and stimulation.

BULBS OF VESTIBULE

The bulbs of the vestibule or vestibular bulbs, surround the openings of the vagina, and urethra. The bulbs consist of two elongated masses of erectile tissue and usually measure about one inch or (2.5cm). Their anterior ends are tapered and have deep surfaces. Superficially, they are covered by the Bulbocavernosus.

The bulbs are between the crura, mentioned above, and the vaginal wall. The paired structures, when aroused, swell with blood, as a male penis will do in arousal, and may double in size.

CORPUS CAVERNOSUM

The corpus cavernosum of the clitoris is paired and is made from sponge-like tissue that is sensitive to stimulation and touch. During a clitoral erection, it fills with blood, like that of the male penis. The term corpus cavernosum simply means a cave-like structure.

Each of the above areas is an essential part of the natal female's body and is to be respected. Having said that, the female may want to explore different areas of her body during a sexual relationship or as an individual! Such exploration, with respect, should be encouraged.

The human body and brain are designed to make and give love, there is nothing dirty or vulgar about it. It is each person's heritage and belief systems, upbringing, religious doctrine, and personal opinions, that create many of the mental boundaries that limit education, not only for adults but the guided information that helps to keep vulnerable people and children safe.

The act of intercourse is how the world and its human beings have come to live in this twenty-first century!

It is the aggression of the act that some people associate with love, sex, and intercourse that causes pain, hurt, anger, spitefulness, and revenge.

Because of the natural nature of sex within human behaviour, it is non-recognition, that sex and intercourse will continue to be taboo, but regardless of taboo, sex will be ongoing within the world societies!

Through the lack of recognition and taboo of the subject, the sex slave trade, vulnerable people, and children will continue to be sexually abused; people will be caught up in domestic violence situations that have roots in sexual abuse, and other sex crimes will continue, with most being committed on innocent people...

Are you now looking from the 'INSIDE OUT?'
YOUR NOTES

....
....
....
....
....
....
....
....
....
....

How To Create a Sexual and Loving Relationship

Where do you now see your assets?
YOUR THOUGHTS

....

....

....

....

....

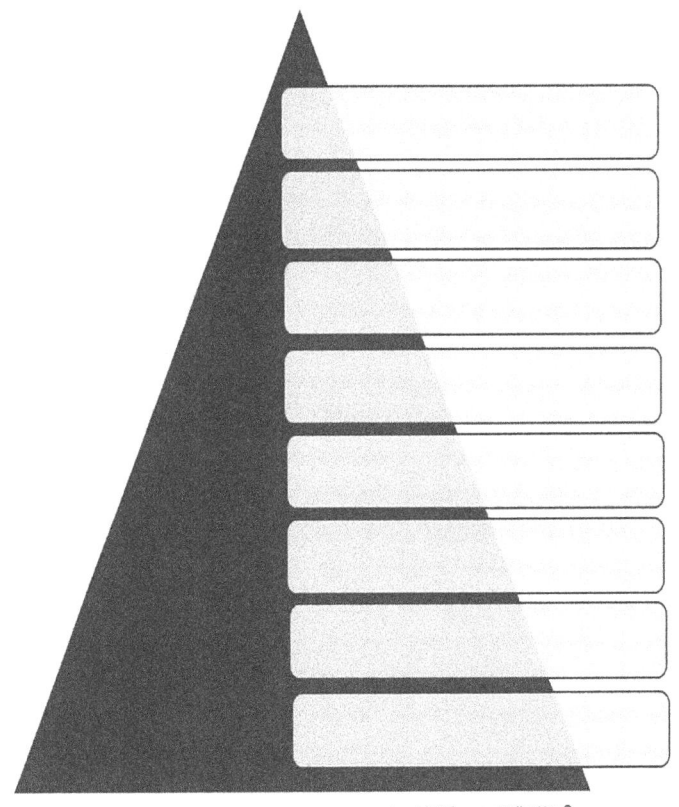

How To Create a Sexual and Loving Relationship

Relationships & Relationship Dynamics

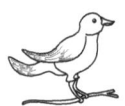 

CHAPTER SEVEN
Relationships & Relationship Dynamics

Starting this chapter on a positive note. Many terms relate to relationships, however, and briefly and within the context of this book, each person who enters a relationship wants to do so, mainly because they have fallen in love, or want to spend more time with somebody they find interesting; they may not be in love at the start of the relationship, but love can blossom!

So, let's expand on relationships. The world is full of relationships, from happy marriages that have lasted over seventy years, and relationships that come together to build charities that support, feed, and bring comfort to people or refugees while their country is under attack from hostile forces!

RELATIONSHIP DYNAMICS
The dynamics within every relationship form allow relationships to flex and grow, change, modify, or become redundant...! When we relate to any relationship,

we are relating to the dynamics at play, the subtleties, undercurrent, forces, and crescendos as in having fun while having committed to and having personal moments in the bedroom!

It is the dynamics of any relationship that play with our senses and emotions, we can feel happy, sad, frustrated, or angry with a situation, and it is all because of different dynamics within the relationship that are either causing us problems or allowing us to enjoy the moments and love the memories...

This book is about you and how you can use this information to add well-being, happiness, and satisfaction to your relationships. When each of us has the extra knowledge, it empowers us, adds to sustainable relationships, and adds quality to our lives. It is the quality of life that is the satisfying dynamic that adds to every relationship the necessary ingredients that allow us to move forward with ease and allow us to reach our full potential.

So, what are the dynamics within relationships?

- ✓ A relationship dynamic implies, that it can be done.
- ✓ Change can be managed which includes effective action is taking place.
- ✓ Regardless of the situation, there is motivation and driving energy to achieve the desired goal.
- ✓ Each partner adds to the motivation, which drives the relationship in a positive direction.
- ✓ The determination and enthusiasm to make changes do not falter but propel forward despite setbacks.
- ✓ Through the energy and enthusiasm of the relationship, momentum is maintained.
- ✓ New ground is found, ideas are sought, and dreams are reached.

Complimentary Dynamics allow relationships to work, so, what are relationship dynamics?

RESPECT

Within any relationship, if respect is missing within the combination of behaviours, and words spoken, it will be difficult to keep the relationship for now and into the future….!

Having said the above, and speaking about your relationship or relationships, how do you see yourself now?

The above is an important question and it is nearly always difficult to dig deeply into your emotions if you are dissatisfied or unhappy! Having said that, you may be happy within your relationship, and you may want to improve on what you currently have.

Please take a little time to think before writing anything down.

....
....
....
....

As you start on this new journey of self-exploration, you are putting yourself on a new expedition of discovery; thinking clearly and with consideration, the journey can become an exciting adventure. If through your journey, you want to include a partner, loved one, or another person to share your experiences, please take some time to think and then keep moving in the positive direction of relationship building.

RELATIONSHIPS

There are many forms of relationships, from a husband and wife to a partner that is legally committed in a formal obligation such as a parenting partner, romantic partner, legal or business partner! Other relationships include friends, acquaintances, customers, and clients, meeting people online, teacher to student, nurse to patient, doctor to nurse, and more. Relationships allow us to connect with other people, which in turn, allows us to function within our own and world communities.

Within any positive and working relationship, there needs to be some main ingredients:

- ✓ Respect
- ✓ Trust

- ✓ If in a legally binding relationship such as marriage, love, and commitment.
- ✓ Honesty
- ✓ Belief
- ✓ Obligation to that relationship, without frets or emotional blackmail.[12]
- ✓ Friendship and enjoyment of each other.
- ✓ Intimacy
- ✓ Loyalty
- ✓ Effective communication
- ✓ Amicable conflict solutions and honesty with decided outcomes.
- ✓ Unplanned acts of kindness and selflessness, and
- ✓ Responsibility for personal choices, caring and consideration to maintain personal health and well-being, caring to aim and reach the same goals for the best benefits for all concerned.

---

[12] Emotional blackmail includes using manipulative behaviours that use guilt, fear, and persuasion, including other people's vulnerabilities which allows the manipulator to control behaviour, choice making and decision making of those people, including children. It involves using pressure to comply with another person's wishes or desires using words, behaviours, including withholding affection, and love to maintain compliance over another person. It typically happens in the breakdown of romantic relationships.

- ✓ If in a temporary relationship, honesty, respect and
- ✓ Prioritisation.

The awareness, practical knowledge, and use of the above considerations will lead to successful relationship building.

BALANCED RELATIONSHIPS – WORKING WITH ACTIVE AND PASSIVE IN RELATIONSHIPS

For a relationship to stay balanced, there needs to be active and passive working.

For instance, though I am a responsible person, for the most part, I rely on my husband to cut the grass, pay the household bills, keep the car registered, and make sure the health funds are financially kept up to date. He, in turn, likes a hot meal at night, a bed with changed clean sheets each week, and occasionally, I keep the ironing up to date – not one of my choice chores, but ironing needs to be done…!

RELATIONSHIPS MATTER

Relationships matter because, as a species, human beings are mainly, social creatures. For example, if you are sick, you go to the doctor; if you want to learn and have recognition for learning, you will find a teaching institution, run by other human beings, who have the knowledge and can pass it on to you, this allows you to acquire the information needed, which allows you to gain the certificate or degree that shows you are competent in that specialisation.

Both previously spoken about scenarios are only achieved because relationships are formed with other people!

PERSONAL RELATIONSHIPS

In personal relationships, you embrace your partner for the person they are, and for the traits and qualities they bring to the relationship. You also respect their needs, and show respect, when and if, they change! Because of love and caring, you may find you adapt to different times, changes, and ideas of your partner! This is all part of working with and adapting to new ideas, progression, growing, expanding your thoughts, and thinking, and the development of the person you will eventually become.

HEALTHY GROWTH

I have been writing books for the last twenty-six years and love every book I write. For instance, the book, 'Devils In Our Food,' took over five years to research and write, and so many times I wanted to walk away from it, but I persevered until I felt, and knew, the book was complete at that time!

My husband is a patient man, he looked on while I struggled, both within myself, researching and continuing with the above book.

And then, after teaching sex education for three years, and knowing there was vital information missing to make sense of how the human body works, I started writing the four children's puberty or sex information books, followed by the parents' support book for their puberty children, and then, I knew I had to write this current book. While doing such a volume of writing, my husband silently supports me, and sometimes, he makes a comment, but for the main part, he is reassuring and forward-thinking... He will give me his ideas, then pause, and we continue the discussion...

Well, after so much writing, my brain needed some much-needed relief, when the writing was done at the end of the day, the dinner was cooked and eaten and then a time to stop. No, television wasn't the answer, but after fourteen years of not painting flower pictures, it was time to put the brush to the canvas again...!

To raise the public consciousness and to start a charity to raise awareness for the need for 'Life Skill Education', for all children, teens, and adults, I am planning to run an art exhibition, connecting art to learning, in fact to 'Life Skill Education!'

Previously, and having taught and counselled young male offenders at a correctional centre, in the United Kingdom, I saw a different side of the confinement and from the eyes and words spoken by some of the young men, knew that change was needed! Most of the young men, not all, were in prison because of minimal offences and offences committed more out of 'peer pressure' rather than vindictiveness, anger, hate, revenge, or greed…!

When young people get into trouble with the law, it is, in many instances, because their relationships within the community in which they live, have broken down!

It would be difficult to do some of the above without the positive relationship I have with my husband who supports me. With the writing, I may run an idea past him for his comments, or I may be in the middle of a painting, and ask, 'What do you think?' Sometimes, he gives constructive criticism, I listen, I modify what I am doing, and sometimes I may try his ideas to see if his suggestions work; this is all part of our relationship!

ACCEPTING OF ANOTHER

In the above, my husband has accepted the choices I am making. He has learnt to embrace the situation, which in turn, allows me to continue my journey.

In all positive relationships, there needs to be reflection. If my husband was to judge or become irritated by what I am doing, it would dampen my enthusiasm, and interfere with my values. Equally so, if I did not encourage him, as a building designer, to continue following his passion to design, and create sustainable, environmentally friendly, and passive homes for people, I too, would be interfering with his long-term goals and values!

Relationships need to be balanced, so, a balanced relationship allows people to genuinely accept their partner and the goals they individually want to achieve.

It is the genuine belief in another person's compassion, and capabilities, along with their qualities, that allows personal relationships to flourish and grow.

DYNAMIC WORKINGS OF RELATIONSHIPS

For family relationships to work effectively there needs to be an active/passive connection between the people within the relationship.

To give you some idea, when jobs need to be done as household work and cutting the grass, there needs to be an equal commitment between those people who have taken on the role to maintain those jobs. By doing so, the household duties are done on time and the flow between home and work is maintained. Such commitments allow each person to keep to their role with family needs being met and a home functioning effectively.

In a scenario, if the only vehicle you have is a horse and cart when one of the wheels falls off the cart, the cartwheel needs to be either replaced or put back on to the cart, then the vehicle can be used as was its first intention!

When, in a relationship, one of the wheels falls off the cart, then there needs to be a solution found to either fix or make amicable adjustments that will modify the relationship and allow it to function in its now modified form.

WORKING TOGETHER

In any relationship, if there is a commitment to work and change, it will incorporate working hard with dedication to make the changes.

When working together, there needs to be the end goal and the commitment to increase the happiness within the relationship. When this is the desired outcome, impossible mountains can be climbed, and great hurdles overcome.

If, however, the outcome is not met, there may be a need for modification to the goal, or it might be a sign that the relationship is incompatible!

SEX AND RELATIONSHIPS

As with intimate adult relationships, sex and togetherness are essential ingredients; sex is the 'mortar between the bricks' that keeps the relationship intact!

The act of sex has an active and passive connection within the intimate times spent enjoying each other's company, and body, and within the intimate sex talk and private moments that people want to spend with each other.

Sex is not a dirty pastime, but a time spent together that allows people to be the people they want to be! Healthy sex releases body tension and relaxes the mind and will allow people to have the pleasantness in life they like and deserve.

With the active and passive approach, when understood, foreplay is a natural part of sexual enjoyment, and it is within these special moments that true love and the enjoyment of another person can be shown.

DISCONNECTED AND DOMINANCE

When a person becomes disconnected in a relationship, it relates to the lack of emotion shown to the other person or people within the relationship.

With some disconnection, it may be due to some form of illness, brought on through a traumatic experience, overuse of alcohol or drugs, or mental illness. Whatever the cause, there may need to be professional medical support or effective counselling sought.

If, while living in a relationship, another person becomes disconnected within the relationship, it was for me, a living hell that I endured.

If, in the relationship, the other person moves from the disconnected state and then assumes a dominant state, and speaking from first-hand experience, the person who disconnects can easily re-connect, becoming the dominant partner. This type of relationship, is again, difficult to accept and live with!

Having either a disconnected or dominant partner within our lives can make life seem like a rollercoaster!

From my own experiences, I never really knew what was going to happen next! Having said that, depending on individual upbringing and personality, people will endure many difficult situations to keep the status quo!

(A note, I speak from first-hand experiences with the above, whilst I hold no malice towards the other person, it becomes a great relief when the experience is over, and the lessons learned...!)

DISENGAGEMENT

Disengagement within any relationship can lead to people looking elsewhere for compatibility and friendship in their lives. Disengagement incorporates both physical and mental abuse, and indeed, all such behaviours mentioned under this heading, including, Disconnected and Dominance, are all areas of abuse on another person.

When a relationship is under stress and a person, or both people become disengaged from within the relationship, it shows there are current problems or problems ahead!

Disengagement within relationships can come about through one of the partner's negative or abusive behaviours, including:

- Physical and mental abuse.
- Consumption of too much alcohol or other mind-altering substances.
- Feeling of little to no value within the relationship and not having personal needs met.
- False assumptions of another's actions.
- Lack of understanding, as in the above, active passive, or one person does all the household chores while another partner sits and watches the other person work...!

(Within this situation, if one partner, through ill health and the lack of physical well-being, is unable to help, there may be a situation of mutual acceptance, even if not spoken about, the agreement is fulfilled which allows the partnership to continue.)

- Financial abuse, withholding money from one partner and making another suffer through the lack of available funds.
- Apathy can be overpowering when a person within any relationship becomes unresponsive to any positive approaches made by the other partner, the relationship, in many instances, has died and may be unretrievable!
- Toxic relationships are described as those relationships that are damaged, unhealthy, or unretrievable. Such relationships may include the following dynamics:
    - Mentally damaging.
    - Unbalanced
    - Destabilizing for individuals or family members.
    - Socially isolating.
    - Emotionally exhausting.
    - Controlling of family members and damaging to human physical and mental health.

There may be more triggers that lead one person in a relationship to become disengaged, if so, you may like to write them down below and possibly speak about them! The choice is yours.

....
....
....
....
....
....
....
....
....
....
....

ALLOSEXUAL, AND ASEXUAL

Most of us can associate with allosexual as it means, those people who find or have experienced sexual attraction at some time in their lives.

Asexual is different in that it can describe two different orientations. In the first instance, asexual may describe a person who has no sexual desires towards any other person. In the second instance, it can describe those people who have little to no sexual desires and yet, they have romantic tendencies towards others, but the tendencies are never fulfilled.

PLATONIC RELATIONSHIPS

Some theorists describe platonic relationships as Basic relationships. Personally, all good relationships are of value, and add a great benefit to our communities.

In all good relationships, there are elements of love, caring, understanding, and non-romantic affection for each other. These relationships are great friendships that stand the test of time. They are there regardless of any financial or material gain, they are indeed great friendships.

Platonic and close-friend relationships, may at times, have a sexual overtone, that may include flirtation, admiration, and attraction, but some boundaries are respected, and the boundaries are not broken regardless of the circumstances that may develop!

CASUAL RELATIONSHIPS

Casual relationships may be described as those types of relationships we have within our working environments, the relationship is good and firm, but only lasts if the employment lasts! Once you have left that employment, the relationship ends.

In some casual relationships, we may confide personal information in a co-worker and hope that the information will never be relayed to another, but it is a casual relationship and should be remembered as that.

Some working, casual relationships may become sexual with an affair taking place, but the deep commitment that makes a relationship endure hardships is not within the makeup of a casual relationship.

In some instances, the relationship that started as a casual relationship may become long-term with other new aspects of the relationship taking over; it becomes a life commitment. The most important part of a casual relationship is that respect for each other and the commitment to change is sincere.

CO-DEPENDENCY

Many co-dependent relationships can be long-term and may describe those relationships that describe personal traits, human interactions between people, caring actions, and or tendencies.

Having said the above and having done a great deal of research for a previous book I have written; the term co-dependency seems to vary over time!

Co-dependency may relate to putting your partner's needs before your own, or mean that you cohabitate with someone to meet different requirements in your life:

- Financial benefits, or
- For convenience and or

- For practical reasons.

If a co-dependent relationship is to survive, it will lack emotional and physical boundaries. Depending on the commitment of the partners in a co-dependent relationship, it may become a loose or flexible relationship...!

Different values, needs, wants, and desires are attached to all relationships, so each partner needs to speak openly about what they want from their co-dependent relationship!

PARTNER

With such a loose term, now used even when speaking of married couples, it implies many suggestions, here are a few:

- Partner, current or otherwise
- Romantic partner
- Sexual partner
- Life partner
- Marriage partner
- Platonic partner

- Partner in love and as discussed earlier in this chapter, there are 'many types of partners!'

MONOGAMOUS RELATIONSHIP

A monogamous relationship means a person will have a relationship with only one person and both have agreed to have only one primary partner, they are romantic, sexual, and may have many common hobbies or interests they enjoy doing together.

This type of relationship is known as a dyadic relationship that is exclusive with firm boundaries and guidelines in place.

OPEN RELATIONSHIPS

An 'open relationship' may have one structured relationship that is permanent but other relationships may co-exist within the partnership of the couple!

The alternative partners may have sexual and loving relationships with other people while knowing that there is always a 'key' person and another partner they can depend on.

In another description, relationships, and friendships can be intimate and loving, but do not engage with romantic or sexual acts!

POLYAMOROUS RELATIONSHIPS

This includes a relation dynamic that has an emotional, romantic, and sexual element, and is for one fixed time only!

POLYGAMOUS RELATIONSHIPS

This relationship is based on agreed guidelines and is related to those involved.

The relationships within the agreement, verbally or written, relate to many sexual relationships at any one time. This may be an agreement between legally married partners and the act of polygamy is recognised by both partners.

REBOUND IN RELATIONSHIPS

The word 'rebound' is often used by people describing another and yet the word in its correct interpretation means, the person who is the object of physical attraction, love, romance, and that partnership has recently ended, or the relationship has changed...

SIGNIFICANT OTHER

A loose interpretation can mean you are a person who has a relationship with another person and is engaging in sexual activities and physical intimacy! You are keeping the relationship under wraps!

There may be other headings that can be used to describe your relationship or relationships! Having now almost finished the book, it is time to do some deep thinking and to determine your next step and the progression you want to take while developing your current relationship or future relationships!

MY FRIEND

At the beginning of the book I mentioned my friend, this story is many years old but has lingered in my mind. We each have different ways of dealing with crisis, change, and the essential growth we each must do if we are going to survive the many traumas we experience in life.

My friend, a beautiful lady, and I had known her for some time before she told me her story. She said, *'My marriage was a disaster, and we were both suffering….!'* I think both people were still in love, but so much had happened during their marriage, at that point, the relationship was irretrievable…! She continues, *'…we had decided to divorce and to move on. It was then that I had as many one-night stands as I could, I think I had about twenty, one after the other, I didn't care!'* She stops, pauses to rethink, then continues with words vaguely like this, *'…I just wanted intimacy, love, and sex; it was the feeling of satisfaction with another person that kept me going and the feeling, I was coping…!'*

We each cannot judge another for the actions they do or take in their lives. Their choices are their choices, and we all do different things at different times!

Stress, change, and life upheavals can have profound effects on us as human beings; each of us will manage these times differently!

When people are in pain, confused, hurt, or are losing their way in life, regardless of their actions, they need support, love, and care shown to them.

We each owe each other, and for human survival, we all need to show empathy and love to others at different times throughout our lives.

As each person travels their life journey, changes will happen. Often, the changes will be unforeseen, and drastic action, to survive both emotionally and physically will need to be taken. When you start to think from the 'inside out,' you are continuing to build your life skills, add strength to your character, and embrace life for what it is offering. Through such actions, you become your survivor.

How To Create a Sexual and Loving Relationship

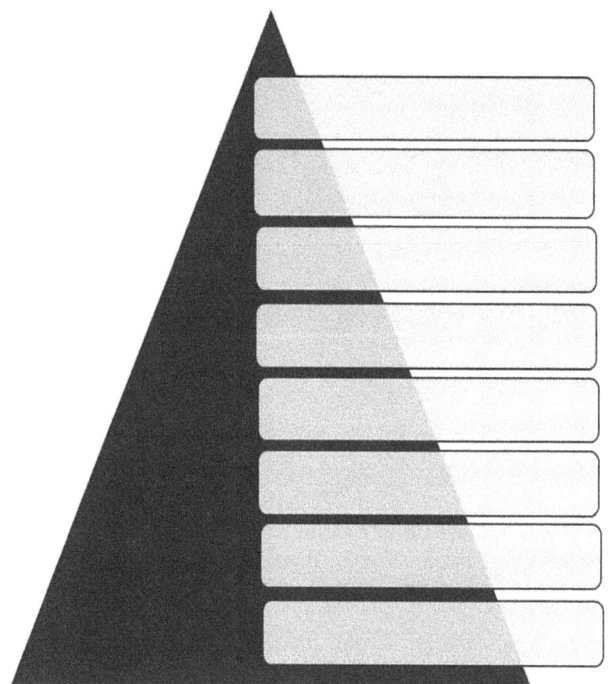

YOUR THOUGHTS

....

....

....

....

....

....

....

....

How To Create a Sexual and Loving Relationship

SUMMING UP – YOUR MIND WHEEL

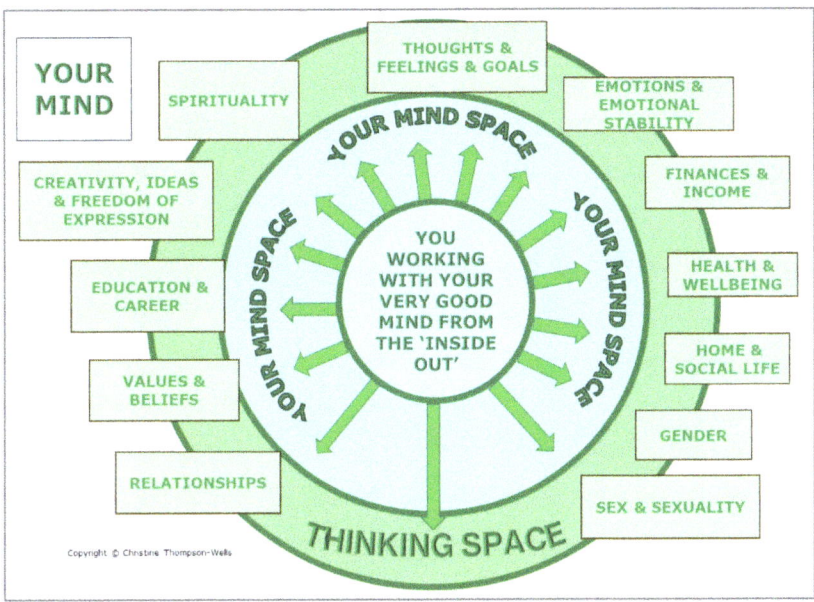

Please take some time to study the above and keep the above when in mind as you work with your Personality Pyramid and reach your goals.

ARE YOU LOOKING FROM THE 'INSIDE OUT'?

How To Create a Sexual and Loving Relationship

ARE YOU LOOKING FROM THE 'INSIDE OUT' OR THE 'OUTSIDE IN?'

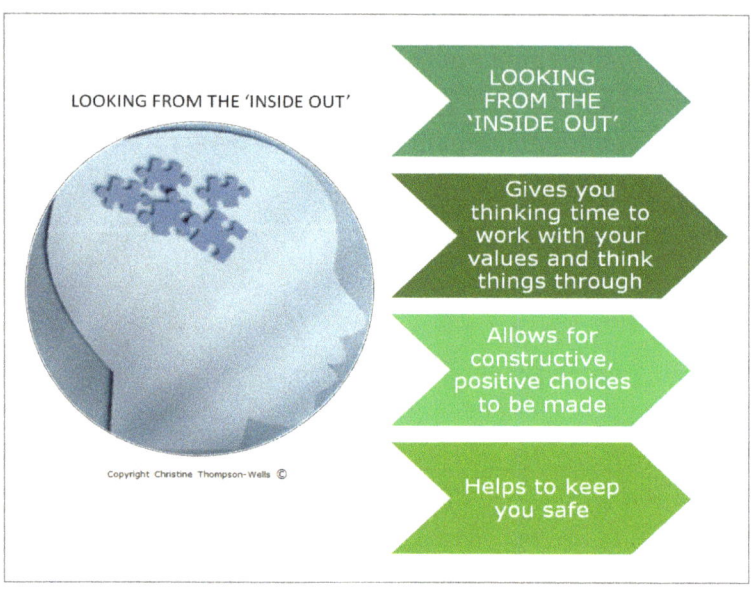

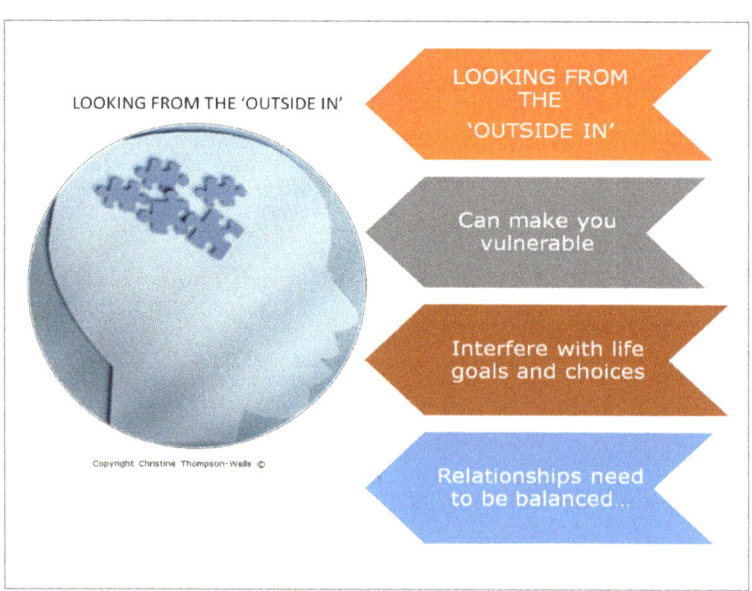

CHAPTER EIGHT
The Ikigai in Each of Us...

I had come to the end of the original book and knew in my heart there was more to do. Throughout writing the course to accompany the book after writing the first and original Sex, Sexuality & Relationships book, it was as though there was an intended message from a source of universal energy. This energy came to my husband in a message from our Goddaughter, Emma. The message spoke about her husband who had been in a 'high-end' very well-paid marketing position with Formula One; he had been made redundant, though having other marketing positions, he wasn't happy...

Currently, he has a position caring for and working with animals! The message spoke about him, the husband finding his ikigai, this information led me to look at my search and the need to constantly write all the books I have written and still more I need to write!

SO, WHAT IS IKIGAI?

When we each reach a point in life and when change is required, we may come to a fork in the road on our life journey, this fork may be a time of making changes that are about fulfilling our destiny with the work that still needs to be done!

WORKING FROM THE 'INSIDE OUT' & NOT THE 'OUTSIDE IN...!'

As I've read through the meaning of ikigai, I was amazed at the information written by an incredibly intuitive and soul-searching writer, according to a study by Michiko Kumano, *'feeling ikigai as described in Japanese usually means the feeling of accomplishment and fulfillment that follows when people pursue their passions.'*

By working from the 'inside out' we can start to evaluate, establish, or re-establish our goals and work towards a brighter, prosperous future. Prosperity is not necessarily about accumulating money and material goods, but it may include inner peace, living and fulfilling dreams, and taking actions that benefit your family and community in good work done!

How To Create a Sexual and Loving Relationship

I feel with all my heart, that the books and courses I now develop are all meant to be part of my life journey, as I have recently said to another woman, *'It is about the journey, not necessarily the financial outcome…!*

FINDING YOUR IKAGAI

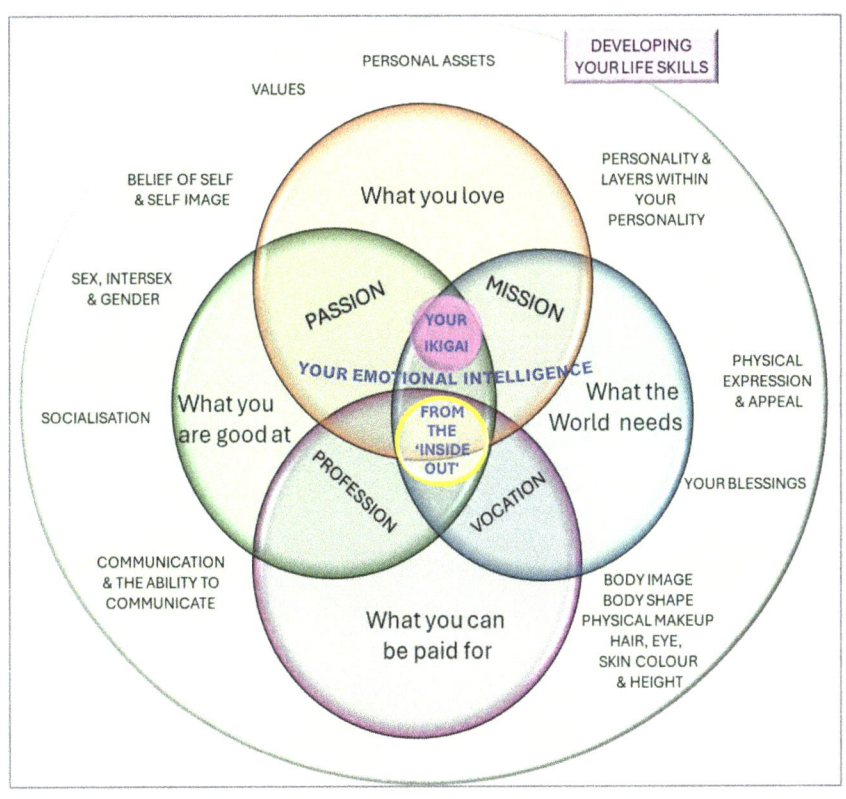

THE JOURNEY YOU'VE TRAVELLED

1. I started the book by introducing you to your **Personality Pyramid** and working down the Pyramid from your Values.
2. You are now aware that your relationships come together through the interaction and interconnection of your **Physiology, Biology, and Psychology**.
3. We then moved on to working with your **Assets** and how your Assets contribute to your relationships.
4. As medically defined at birth, we are either born as **Natal Male**, **Natal Female**, or **Intersex**. How we wish to define ourselves as adults is a personal choice.
5. Defining **sexuality** is through identifying the **gender** we each have within our personalities and is too, a matter of personal choice.
6. **Hormones** play an essential role in, not only how our body and brain work, but also within the sexual relationships we each may have.

7. When our sex hormones are charged with high octane, we may be attracted to **'eye candy'**, and not all 'eye candy' is what it appears to be on the outside...!
8. **Respect** is a fundamental concept within the book's information. Regardless of the length of time, respect must always be the biggest part of any relationship.
9. The human **genitals** are sensitive areas within the male and female body and should be treated with respect, love, and care always.
10. The **dynamics** within relationships vary and change through time.
11. There are **many types** of human relationships (both positive and negative) working within our communities, each has its uniqueness.
12. Finding your **Ikigai** is a personal journey; finding your ikigai will allow you to extend your talents, grow positively from the experience, and support you in working from your 'inside out.'

Loving, sexual relationships are built with respect and trust.

ONCE WE KNOW THE REASON WHY, WE ARE BETTER EQUIPPED TO UNDERSTAND WHY CHANG HAPPENS...!

How To Create a Sexual and Loving Relationship

SOME OF MY BOOKS

With over sixty books written, here are some of Christine's titles available at www.how2books.com.au and through major worldwide book outlets.

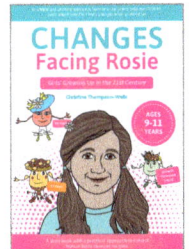

The 'Changes,' series for children and young people are written for ages, 9-11 and 11-14 years.

The books are a gentle way of taking a child on the journey of identifying how all children will go from being a child into adulthood.

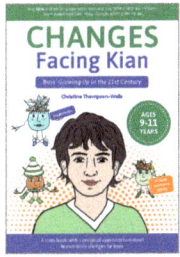

Each book has a six-chapter beginning which includes an adventure story, with each story taking place in a different location around the world. The countries included are Bologna, Italy, Scotland, Ireland, and Australia.

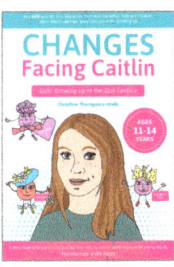

To allow the young person to easily identify with the story and characters, not forgetting the hormone journey they are on, we have included the correct hormone name in the 9-11-year-old books and have identified the hormones by giving them hats. 'Hormones With Hats,' each hormone has a different hat, and this makes for instant recall and recognition by the child.

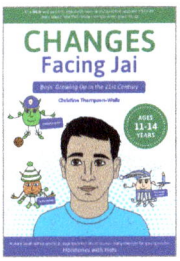

We continue this theme, however, in the 11-14-year-old books, the hormone name and the chemical symbol for the related hormone are shown.

Learning about the body is part of life skill education and needs to be embraced for self-sustainability, well-being, and good health.

The second part of each book is a workbook that allows for parents, family, teachers, and those people speaking on the subject in community groups, to interact with the child or students.

If you have bought the puberty books and you are a school or community group, we will provide your school or group with a secure, FREE online, puberty education package.

The secure links, once contacted at the below email address, will be sent back to you at the email address you have provided. Please email: admin@fullpotentialtraining.com.au.

The links are valid for 30 days, so please have your dates secured before emailing us.

All books meet the United Kingdom and Australian Curriculum National Standards.

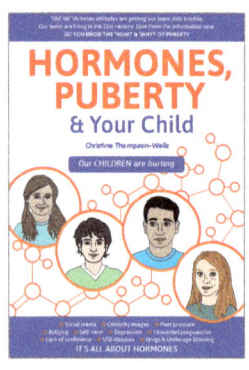

For those parents who want to read and become familiar with this latest information, we have written and published the supporting book for you, 'Hormones, Puberty & Your Child.'

How To Create a Sexual and Loving Relationship

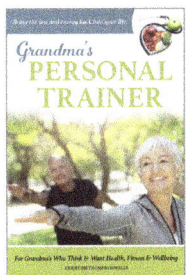

Age is but a number! As I am a grandmother and love to keep fit, with the support of a personal trainer, I have written this book. Through doing a few exercises each day, I keep my body and mind healthy. I have drawn line illustrations that show simple daily exercises, some sitting in a chair, such exercises can help to maintain body and muscle strength while exercising helps to keep your immune system healthy.

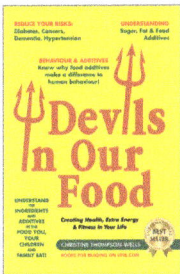

A book, mentioned in this book, Devils in Our Food, which took over five years to write, is an informative book that alerts us to the poisonous additives going into many food products in this twenty-first century.

Many of the additives mentioned are causing cancer and other health problems and conditions, not only in older adults but also in children and babies. At the start of the research for Devils in Our Food, there were just over three hundred additives mentioned on the Australian government website, there are now over ten thousand going into the world manufactured food supply.

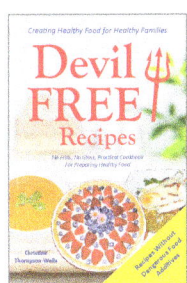

Devil Free Recipes is just as it says on the cover. Feeling exasperated by the additives now going into everyday foods, like breakfast cereal, it was time to give some solutions and here they are. Prepare your recipes and know exactly what ingredients you and your family are eating.

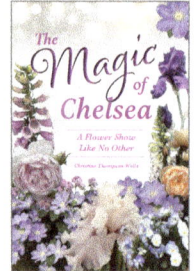
Before going to university and becoming a teacher and writer, I trained as a florist in London, United Kingdom. It is my love of flowers that drives me back to the United Kingdom each year to collect the information that allows us to publish this beautiful book of over 270 photographs and over 170 pages of detailed information on the displays, different exhibits, new varieties of blooms and more.

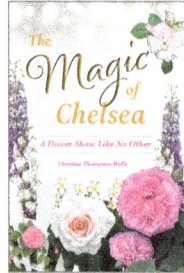
Our publication of The Magic of Chelsea from 2023, is still available.

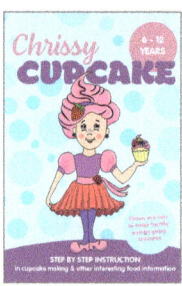
Learning, as a child, about the dangers in the kitchen, while making delicious cupcakes is, again, life skill building. It is the magical moments spent with our children that helps to keep them safe as adults. Learning about adding healthy ingredients to baking, is healthy eating, and all children need to know about the food they eat!

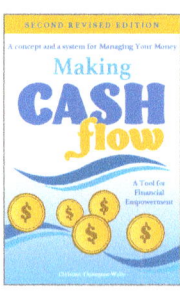
This book never reduces in its popularity. It sells constantly throughout the world and why? The book incorporates many good money management ideas and ideas that don't go out of date. It is the psychology of money management that empowers the reader and the words on the pages.

It was managing a business through a recession that inspired me to write 'Making Cash Flow.' After all, even during a recession, the same amount of money is in the community, but the money is going in another direction – this is money psychology! It's understanding that money is inert, and is of no value, it is the value we, and within our human minds, that we as individuals place on money, that makes it valuable!

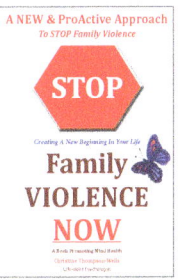

It is the hidden horror of family violence that people don't want to speak about. Sadly, it happens in many homes around the world.

The book has been written from personal experiences and will support those people who want to make changes in their lives.

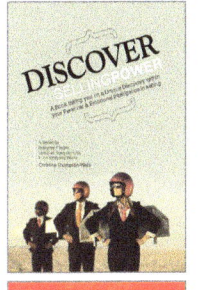

Having had businesses selling products to the public, there are certain considerations and 'knowing how to sell' that lead to a successful 'close' of the sale!

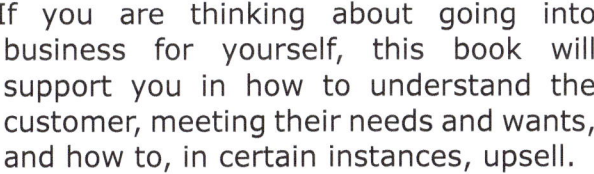

If you are thinking about going into business for yourself, this book will support you in how to understand the customer, meeting their needs and wants, and how to, in certain instances, upsell.

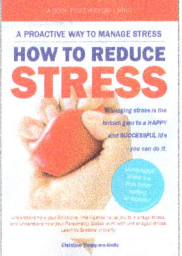

There are many stressors in modern life, and it is knowing how to manage your health and well-being that allows you to successfully navigate the different situations you daily face while doing the jobs that need to be done!

From running businesses, managing family life, and working within dysfunctional relationships, this is all part of what many people face daily. From my own experiences, I write the books and I relate to and have experienced all I write about!

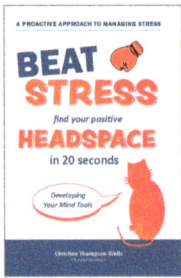

I was inspired to write this book, and strangely enough, I have written the book from the perspective of a cat. That is not meant as a derogatory comment, but the stress, we are nearly all experience, is perpetrated and added to by the way we see every situation.

Beating stress can be done; it is the negative mindset we mentally develop that adds to every stressful situation. Managing stress is knowing, 'How to Manage Stress!'

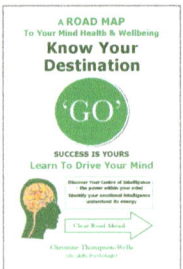

Every situation can be overcome, this was the inspiration for this book. We can grow from each, of what appears to be a negative situation, and we can learn from the experiences, though at the time, we may feel the experience is insurmountable!

From losing all material belongings to starting again and becoming successful, it is achievable through clear thinking, writing down, and keeping to your daily goals, you will surprise yourself at the achievements you can accomplish.

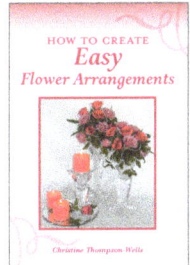

From florist to teacher and then to writer! All of this has been possible through hard work and determination. Because I believe that all people can learn and fulfil their dreams and many people want to learn about flower arranging and some, from this book alone, have started their own small businesses. This book guides you through the early stages of learning this life skill and from me, I can truly say, in many instances, the skills of knowing how to arrange flowers has been a financial lifeline!

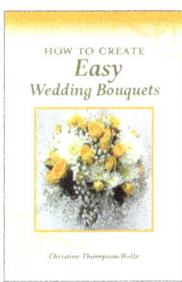

Again, I have written this book that allows you to learn how to construct wedding bouquets and from this knowledge, if you start small, you may eventually start a business in exclusive wedding bouquet and designs.

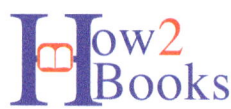

www.ingramcontent.com/pod-product-compliance
Lightning Source LLC
Chambersburg PA
CBHW062034290426
44109CB00026B/2630